You can
SLEEP
SOUNDLY
EVERY
NIGHT
without drugs

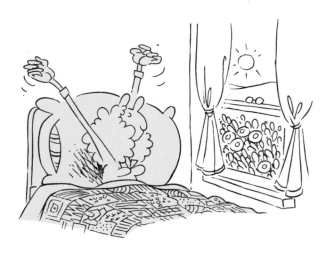

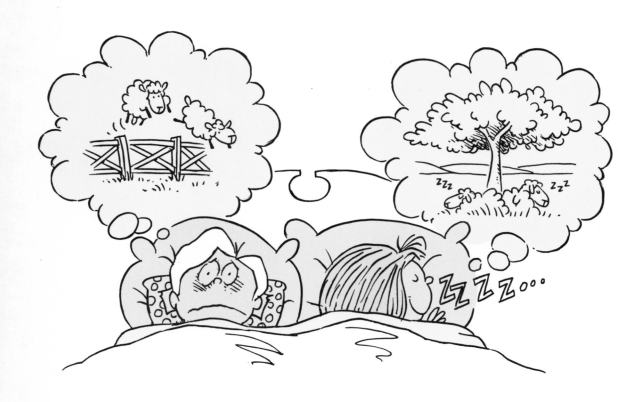

You can SLEEP SOUNDLY EVERY *NIGHT* *without drugs*

A PROVEN SELF-HELP PROGRAM

DR IAN BRIGHTHOPE
WITH
PETER FITZGERALD

BAY BOOKS
Sydney and London

ABOUT THE AUTHORS

Dr Ian Brighthope is President of the Australian College of Nutritional Medicine and lectures internationally on health topics.

Peter Fitzgerald is a Melbourne freelance writer who specialises in medical and consumer subjects for the popular market.

Published by Bay Books, 61–69 Anzac Parade, Kensington, NSW 2033

Copyright text © Peter Fitzgerald with Dr Ian Brighthope

National Library of Australia
Card number and ISBN 1 86256 331 4

Cartoons by Brian Kogler
Illustrations by Greg Gaul

Designed by Susan Kinealy

Typesetting by Savage Type Pty Ltd, Brisbane
Printed in Singapore by Toppan Printing Co.

BB 89

CONTENTS

The real doctor is the doctor within.

Most doctors know nothing of this science and yet it works so well.

ALBERT SCHWEITZER

INTRODUCTION

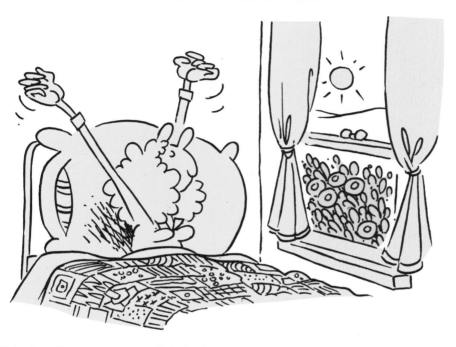

With the disappearance of their insomnia, most people experience an improvement in their mood, happiness and ability to cope — and a belief that there is light at the end of the tunnel — that life can be lived with an improved sense of wellbeing, achievement of goals, ambitions. In other words, they feel that life is truly worth living.

Sleep is essential for the rejuvenation of every cell in the body, particularly the cells of the nervous system. When we sleep, all our systems slow down, giving the body a chance to repair itself. Other functions of sleep, such as dreaming, are important in restoring psychological balance.

The amount of sleep we need is like many other aspects of life in that the requirements vary from person to person. Individual differences in diet and nutrition occur, individual differences in requirements for love and affection also occur, and so do individual differences in requirements for sleep.

Age also appears to play a role. Babies and children require much more sleep than do adults. The average teenager and young adult generally requires about eight to nine hours of good quality sleep each night. As we enter our sixties and seventies, the requirements for sleep become less and many people seem to need only five to seven hours sleep a night.

When we sleep all our systems slow down, giving the body a chance to repair itself.

7

Insomnia

The body is a complex chemical factory and many influences can cause a disturbance in it.

As will become clear while reading this book, the body is a complex chemical factory and many influences can cause a disturbance in it. When such disturbances occur, insomnia may result.

Insomnia is the most common disorder of sleep. It is the inability to sleep or the inability to attain satisfactory sleep during normal sleeping hours. It includes the inability to get off to sleep, to stay asleep and the problem of early morning awakening with its attendant inability to return to normal sleep. It also includes really restless and disturbed sleep in which the person continually wakes throughout the night, often in a state of anxiety or panic.

These disorders of sleep usually have an effect on a person's day-to-day functioning and can result in them feeling tired, depressed, tense and unable to work or concentrate on their normal daily activities.

Some experts suggest that disordered sleep and insomnia can be related to daytime napping or changes in overall sleep habits. However, there is no good evidence for this. In fact, a short daytime nap can often contribute to an improvement in one's health and the ability to carry out daily activities. This can be seen in the Mediterranean countries, where a daytime siesta for one or two hours is routinely taken.

How big is the problem?

It is difficult to evaluate how many people have troubles with sleeping and sleep disorders, but it is estimated that approximately 30 per cent of the population will complain of insomnia of some sort while 20 per cent will seek help for it.

It is estimated that approximately 30 per cent of the population will complain of insomnia of some sort while 20 per cent will seek help for it.

Complaints of sleep disturbance increase with increasing age. They also increase with increasing levels of anxiety and mild depression and these problems can be related not only to psychological factors but also to social, cultural and dietary factors.

Dietary factors probably play a more important role than has been previously realised. In fact, we will show later in this book how dietary factors can be manipulated to improve sleeping patterns.

Sleeping drugs

Drugs such as hypnotics and sedatives are effective initially for people who suffer from insomnia and disorders of sleep but they actually reduce the rapid eye movement (REM) sleep as well as reducing the quality of sleep.

They also become very quickly tolerated, and as a result the doses of the drugs have to be increased or the drug changed to another type of medication.

The use of a number of sleeping drugs over a period of time produces a marked decrease of both REM sleep and non-REM sleep. When the drug or drugs are withdrawn, there is a rebound increase in both types of sleep. This can again produce disturbances.

If you're taking sleeping drugs or tranquillisers to aid sleep, it's desirable to continue them until the program in this book starts to take effect. You will notice this by falling asleep more easily and staying asleep. Waking refreshed is another sign that the program outlined in this book is working. Only then is it the right time to start reducing the drugs. You should do this under the supervision of an experienced physician if the sleep disorder was complicated by psychological or medical problems.

The best way to stop medication is slowly, over a four to six week period, reducing the medication by approximately a quarter to a third of the dose every ten days.

The best way to stop medication is slowly, over a four to six week period, reducing the medication by approximately a quarter to a third of the dose every ten days.

What causes insomnia?

There are many factors and causes which can contribute to insomnia and the inability to obtain an adequate quality and quantity of sleep. These causes can be divided into a number of major categories.

1. PSYCHOLOGICAL CAUSES

- Anxiety.
- Disorders of mood — mania and depression.
- Fear of dying while asleep.
- Schizophrenia.
- Unexpressed anger or resentment.

2. MEDICAL CAUSES

- Any painful or discomforting disorder.
- The irritable bowel syndrome.
- Hardening of the arteries.
- Infections.
- Hypertension (high blood pressure).
- Heart disorders.
- Asthma.
- Anaemia.
- Cramping.
- Arthritis.
- Parkinson's disease.
- Pregnancy.
- Premenstrual syndrome.
- Sleep apnoea.
- Hyperventilation syndrome.
- Restless legs syndrome.
- Diabetes.
- Urinary frequency.
- Narcolepsy with cataplexy.

3. DRUG RELATED CAUSES

- Medical drugs and other prescribed medications.
- Paradoxical insomnia — insomnia caused by so-called sedatives.

- Legalised drugs including tea, coffee, chocolate, cola drinks, caffeinated beverages, tobacco and alcohol.
- Recreational drugs including cocaine, glue-sniffing, marijuana.

4. *SOCIAL CAUSES*

- Arguing between family and with friends.
- Financial problems.
- Watching excessively exciting TV programs before going to bed.
- Over-stimulation at night-time generally.
- Sleeping or napping excessively during the day.

5. *DIETARY CAUSES*

- Consuming excessively large meals before bed.
- Excessive hunger.
- Food allergies and chemical intolerances.
- Food additives, especially sugar.
- Functional reactive hypoglycaemia.
- Obesity.
- Nutritional deficiencies.
- Caffeine.

6. *PHYSICAL CAUSES*

- Noise.
- Bright lights.
- Sleeping in an over-heated or under-heated room.
- Poor ventilation.
- An uncomfortable bed with too few or too many bedclothes.

1

The thirty-five most-asked QUESTIONS ABOUT SLEEP

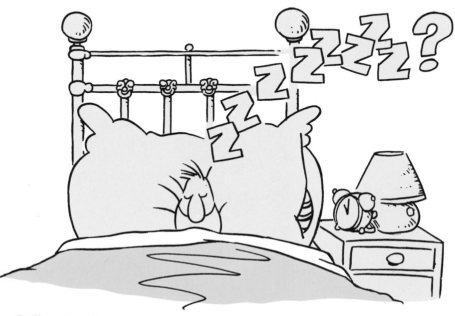

Why is sleep necessary?

A lack of sleep is probably blamed for most people's irritability and tension. Sleep is essential for the rejuvenation of every cell in the body, particularly the brain and the nervous system. It's essential for the stimulation of the growth and restorative processes of the body. Other functions, including dreaming, are also important in restoring good health and psychological balance.

Sleep is essential for the rejuvenation of every cell in the body, particularly the cells of the nervous system.

Does sleep affect your life-span?

People who tend to live longer and have fewer illnesses generally have between seven and eight hours sleep a night — no more and no less.

What controls sleep?

Sleep research indicates that our brain and body need to switch off at night and that there is a biological clock mechanism in all organisms, including humans, which controls this.

We need to spend one-third of our lives in an altered state of consciousness — that is, sleep. Human beings sleep for long stretches at a time whereas most other animals sleep for short stretches and then awaken.

How many people suffer from insomnia?

One in five people suffer from a severe sleep disorder of some sort. Many of them resort to expensive drugs in the hope of getting a good night's sleep. A simple change in diet and lifestyle is all that is needed to cure insomnia and sleep disorders in most people.

Does insomnia affect our work?

The brain and nervous system tend to slow down and not to work as well after a bad night's sleep. Insomniacs find it hard to work effectively and efficiently during the day.

Does sleep affect my looks?

Proper regular sleep benefits not only the mind and brain but produces an improvement in the overall condition of the skin, hair, eyes and general bodily functions including appetite and bowel habits.

I think I sleep well but I feel and look tired. Why?

The appearance of an insomniac is one of puffiness around the eyes and dark circles under the eyes. This can often reflect an underlying illness, especially allergy. You should attempt to find out what it is.

What happens if I have too much sleep?

Over-sleeping, or excessive sleep, causes an overall slowing down of the body and the mind including physical and mental sluggishness, depression and a lack of vitality.

What are the effects of sleep deprivation?

The deprivation of sleep results in a reduction of psychological and intellectual abilities of the individual. This process can be seen clearly in the activities of terrorists who, as practised interrogators, have found that the surest way to extract information from prisoners is to deprive them of sleep. For example, after two nights without sleep people show an increase in anxiety and irritability, slurring of speech and a disorientation with respect to time and space. They find it difficult to recall the time, date and place where they are. Misperceptions of a visual nature also occur and, although these are not hallucinations, they can be quite frightening and misleading all the same.

It's probable, from the findings of research, that to have less than five hours of sleep a night is actually dangerous to your health.

The increased irritability from sleep deprivation is manifested by an increased reaction to any mild stimulus which can cause anxiety, weeping, depression, and an increased sensitivity to painful stimuli.

What is the minimum amount of sleep I can have?

It's probable, from the findings of research, that to have less than five hours of sleep a night is actually dangerous to your health.

Can relaxation or meditation affect my insomnia?

The brain usually cannot switch off during waking states. However, individuals who have learned how to relax deeply or meditate often find that a period of meditation freshens them and reduces their sleep requirements. The meditative state is an altered state of consciousness which is reflected in changes in the electronic brain wave patterns recorded by EEG machines.

It has been claimed that it is possible to relax the whole body's musculature while awake, but never the brain. However, yogis and experienced meditators would disagree. They believe that the meditative state is an altered state of consciousness which is neither awake nor asleep. Meditators generally claim they have better quality sleep and need less of it.

People who meditate generally claim they have better quality sleep and need less of it.

**A PATIENT CONNECTED TO AN EEG MACHINE
TO RECORD BRAIN WAVES**

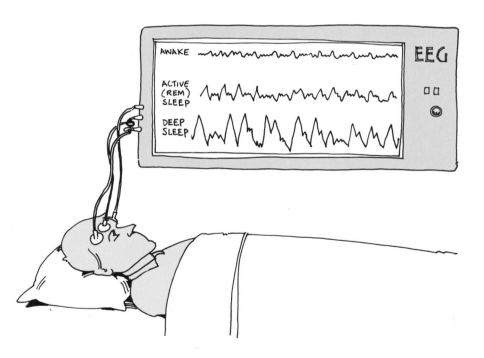

Brain waves from the same person when awake (top), dreaming (middle) and when in deep sleep.

Dream sleep or Rapid Eye Movement (REM) sleep is essential for mental and physical health.

What about the relationship between stress and sleep?

During our wakeful hours, there's always an elevated level of the stress hormone adrenaline in our bloodstream. Adrenaline has many effects on our system including increasing our pulse rate, heart beat, sweating and alertness. In excess, it can actually cause heart palpitations, anxiety, sweating and tremors.

Excessive adrenaline can reduce the production of new tissues in the body. It can also slow down the rate of healing. In conjunction with the production of other stress hormones in excess, including cortisone, it can result in degenerative disease. Therefore, at some time we need to shut off the stress hormones, adrenaline and cortisone, so that our body can generate new tissue and repair old tissue effectively.

It's during sleep that the production of stress hormones is shut down and this regeneration occurs. It also allows the body's glands to manufacture and store hormones for times of need.

Does sleep benefit immunity and healing?

Other benefits of sleep and perhaps even those of deep relaxation states, including meditation, are the mobilisation of fatty tissues and the modulation and improvement of functioning of the immune system.

A persistent lack of sleep and chronic wakefulness with tension results in slowed healing processes and diminution of the functioning of the immune system with resulting increased numbers of infections. For example, colds and flu become more frequent. An increased tendency towards inflammation of the tissues such as arthritis, dermatitis and colitis also occurs.

What is the economic impact of insomnia?

Sleeping pills are one of the most widely prescribed drugs, costing the country millions of dollars each year.

Insomnia is probably the most common complaint brought to doctors and certainly sleeping pills are one of the most widely prescribed drugs, costing the country millions of dollars a year. Approximately one in five people suffer from some form of insomnia. That is, in Australia, approximately three million people fall into this category.

What is the best time to sleep?

It's far better to sleep when it's dark and to be awake in the daylight, as the quality of sleep during the night hours appears to be better. People who work at night and sleep during the day tend to have more psychological problems, some of which may be related to the time of their sleeping.

Why should we be exposed to sunlight?

A hormone called melatonin is produced by the pineal gland in the brain during the hours of darkness and when the eyes are exposed to darkness or closed. It's this hormone which enables animals to hibernate. How-

14

ever, in the case of humans, it causes depression and lassitude rather than hibernation. Melatonin production is switched off when full spectrum sunlight falls on the eye's retina.

It has been found that sunlight is helpful in some forms of depression and it may be that in some depressed people the presence of sunlight reduces melatonin production, and thus reduces the depression.

Active individuals who spend time outdoors tend to suffer from less depression than people who are cooped up in offices, factories and homes all day.

Can depression be helped with sleep?

It's been suggested that depressed people who suffer from insomnia and who go to bed late and rise late should try to break that habit by awakening earlier and exposing themselves to the early morning sunlight for half an hour to an hour. Going to bed earlier also helps to break this cycle.

Is regular sleep important?

Regular sleep is the most beneficial. You should aim to go to bed at the same time every night and to arise at the same time every morning. An occasional sleepless night does very little harm and should not be worried about.

Regular sleep is the most beneficial. You should aim to go to bed at the same time every night and to arise at the same time every morning.

Can herbs and vitamins influence insomnia?

Certain nutritional supplements help to induce sleep and relaxation. These are discussed in Chapters 7 and 8.

What other things can be done to assist sleep?

Hot baths are very relaxing and are useful just before going to bed. Meditation and visualisation can also be useful as can hypnotherapy. Exercising in the morning or afternoon is an excellent way of producing a state of pleasant fatigue which helps induce a good night's sleep. However, you should not exercise late in the evening and just before going to bed.

Exercising in the morning or afternoon is an excellent way of inducing a good night's sleep.

Can exercise keep me awake?

The immediate effects of exercise are to stimulate the system and this is not satisfactory before going to bed because the stimulation will keep you awake.

The later effects of exercise are relaxation and fatigue if the exercise is sufficient. This, of course, will help produce a good night's sleep.

Walking and swimming are the best exercises although callisthenics and light stretching exercises, yoga, Tai Chi and so on are all good methods of exercising.

Midnight waking — What can I do?

Waking in the middle of the night is sometimes a problem and it's better to get up and read a book than to lie in bed tossing and turning.

Eating, drinking, smoking and television are bad if you wake in the middle of the night. The best advice is simply to read a book or do some very light stretches to relax the muscles.

Take a complex of tryptophan, vitamins, minerals and herbs for insomnia before retiring. This will ensure a sound sleep.

Does music help insomnia?

Over-stimulation from loud noises, including music, is not a good thing late at night. However, soft, soothing and relaxing music can definitely help sleep.

Can I take drugs or medicines to help?

One basic rule is not to take sleeping pills, tranquillisers or anti-depressants except in times of great stress, and only for very short periods of time.

One basic rule is not to take sleeping pills, tranquillisers or antidepressants except for a very short time and only if it's absolutely necessary to overcome a particularly stressful period. Drugs induce unnatural sleep which is not beneficial and in the long term are definitely harmful. They can cause further depression of the nervous system and this chemical depression only aggravates insomnia and psychological symptoms.

Should the amount of sleep bother me?

Another basic rule is not to worry about how much sleep you get as this only creates further stress. Instead, follow the basic rules outlined in this book. Try to have between seven and eight hours sleep every night.

What do hypnotic drugs do?

Many insomniacs find the use of sedatives, or hypnotic drugs, an unsatisfactory solution to their sleep disorder. All hypnotic drugs, including chloral hydrate, the barbiturates, and the benzodiazepines, will drastically reduce the dreaming or REM phase of sleep.

However, tryptophan/vitamin/herbal complexes actually improve the quality of sleep and enhance both the deep and REM phases of sleep. These natural complexes are not habit forming and quickly promote a return to a normal, healthy sleep-wake cycle. If necessary they can be taken safely for months at a time.

Why is dreaming necessary?

Dreaming is absolutely essential for mental as well as physical wellbeing.

Deprivation of REM, or dream sleep, results in increased irritability, anxiety or tension during the waking hours and this will eventually result in severe psychological depression. Dreaming is absolutely essential for mental as well as physical wellbeing.

Can I become addicted or tolerant to sleeping drugs?

Tolerance eventually develops to sleep-inducing drugs. This happens after a variable period — from four to twenty-four weeks of taking them. When tolerance to drugs occurs, the drug either has to be changed or the dosage increased. By increasing the dose of an hypnotic drug, daytime sedation occurs the next day and this can often be severe and associated with fatigue, a hangover-like feeling and mental depression.

What happens if I want to stop taking sleeping tablets?

The withdrawal of a hypnotic drug often results in a rebound effect with more severe insomnia than before. The withdrawal of a drug with its rebound effect and then the addition of another hypnotic drug with its possible side effects can be devastating. Psychiatric and sometimes neurological problems eventually surface.

The replacement of one hypnotic drug with another can result in severe psychological disturbances. Withdrawal from hypnotic drugs is often accompanied by a rebound increase in REM sleep with vivid dreams and fantasies. These excessively vivid dreams further disturb sleep. This withdrawal syndrome can be partially or totally alleviated with tryptophan/vitamin/herbal complexes.

How long does it take to get back to normal?

A normal sleeping pattern may take up to two months to be re-established after the cessation of sleeping drugs. Hypnotic or sleeping drugs have a profound effect on the brain's biochemistry. This is not good in the insomniac whose brain biochemistry is already disturbed.

What's the best advice for someone who can't sleep?

The most important advice you can give to a chronic insomniac is to look for the underlying causes for their insomnia and then carefully manage those causes. The use of naturally occurring hypnotic substances found in foods and herbs should be the treatment of first choice.

The most common causes of insomnia and sleep disturbances are anxiety, depression, conditions producing pain, heart failure, lung disease, bladder problems, dietary factors and drugs including sugar, tea, coffee, chocolate, cola drinks, nicotine, alcohol, marijuana, cocaine and medicines.

What are the most useful, safe substances for insomnia?

Probably the most useful nutrient supplement to treat insomnia is tryptophan. This is also useful in the treatment of depression, anxiety and drug-related insomnia. Some studies have found it to be useful in seventy per cent of insomniacs and equally as effective as the tricyclic antidepressant drugs for treating mild to moderate depression.

Tryptophan works by being converted in the brain to a chemical called serotonin. This is a major messenger chemical which travels between nerve cells in the brain relaying information controlling sleep, appetite, mood and sexual appetite (libido). Tryptophan requires an enzyme and vitamin B6 for its conversion to serotonin so these must also be available.

Are dietary supplements safe?

The use of dietary supplements is a totally natural way of obtaining a better sleep. There are no harmful side effects and the supplements are not habit forming or addictive. Taken in the doses recommended, they are safe and often provide beneficial spin-offs. For example, relief of pain or tension, improvement of memory and concentration.

Should I take supplements with meals?

No! Tryptophan should be taken either on an empty stomach or with fruit juice about one hour before retiring. It should not be taken with protein-containing foods because these compete for absorption with one another. Protein-containing foods are milk and dairy products, meat, fish, legumes and eggs.

What can I do about disturbing dreams?

Persistent and bizarre dreams may indicate an underlying psychological disorder and require evaluation by a psychiatrist. However, certain medications may also cause disturbing dreams. If the dreams are transient, the tryptophan complexes may be most useful. Excessively high doses of vitamin B6 or the amino acid called methionine may cause vivid dreaming.

2

How to get
A GOOD NIGHT'S SLEEP

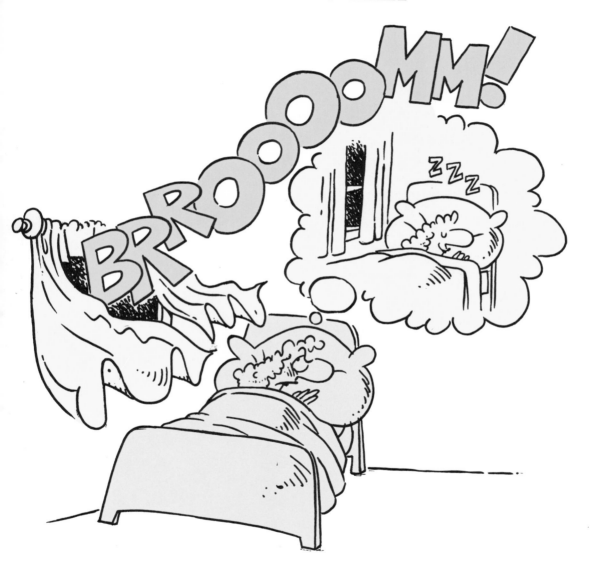

It's commonsense, but often overlooked, that the bedroom should be well designed and comfortable for a good night's sleep. However, when people who suffer from insomnia are asked about their bedroom, many often have an obvious problem in this area which is contributing to their sleeplessness. Take the case of Betty.

Betty's Story

The noise was so great in the dirty, noisy factory environment where Betty spent twelve hours a day that she had to wear ear muffs most of the time. Betty, a twenty-six-year-old factory process worker, discovered that the pleasantly quiet environment of her bedroom at night was ideal for sound slumber once she drifted off.

However, she also discovered that if she played soft music before going to bed, it made it easier and quicker for her to get to sleep. The soft music probably acted as some form of balancing force to the loud and irritating noises she experienced through the day.

It must be emphasised that there's no one single cause for a sleepless night and many factors play a role, including the comfort of the bed, the temperature of the bedroom, your state of mind, external noises in the environment and so on. In this chapter, I will try to cover as many aspects of the bed and the bedroom as possible so that you can make the necessary changes to help your sleep patterns.

Your bedroom

Again, it may seem obvious that the bedroom should be in part of the house that is quiet and away from noisy street frontages and as far as possible from busy highways and industrial areas. Of course, in an area where planes are taking off and landing, the location of the bedroom in the house is irrelevant.

The bedroom must be comfortable, well-situated, and well-ventilated with open windows allowing the inflow of fresh air.

If you live in an inner city area, where the air is highly polluted and there's a lot of traffic, it's wise to perhaps close the windows and shut out the stale and polluted air and noise. It would be better to shift the bedroom to the other side of the house away from the traffic. It's important that the bedroom should be situated away from the living quarters of the house to avoid noise created by other members of the household.

The temperature of the bedroom should be around twenty-one degrees Celsius. If it's too cold, sleep is disturbed and of course, if it's excessively hot, then restless nights ensue.

Bed and bedclothes

Most importantly, the bed should be comfortable with a firm base and mattress that doesn't sag. The pillows should also be comfortable and not excessively hard or soft. They should be of cotton filling if you suffer any form of inhalant allergy or nasal stuffiness.

The bedclothes should be made of cotton and be no more than one sheet and a woollen blanket as an over-cover. Too many blankets, doonas and eiderdowns lying on top of you will certainly maintain warmth, but at the expense of comfort.

The only purpose of a heavy weight of bedclothes on the sleeping individual is a false sense of security. In very cold climates, a light doona is all that's required to maintain even body warmth.

Fresh air

I cannot over-emphasise the value of fresh air for good health. This is especially so for insomniacs who tend to breathe very shallowly when they are asleep. As a result of shallow breathing, they tend to rebreathe their own stale air. This results in a heavy hangover feeling the next morning.

The circulation of fresh air throughout the bedroom at night is one of the best ways of ensuring a fresh, wakeful morning. Over-sleeping is just as bad for your health as under-sleeping, especially if you over-sleep in an airtight room without the health-giving properties of good clean air.

Some people find the presence of an air ioniser in the room at night with them helps to improve the quality of their sleep. It's worth considering this as an investment for someone who does have insomnia, particularly associated with upper airway symptoms such as hay fever, nasal stuffiness, sinusitis or headaches.

The circulation of fresh air throughout the bedroom at night is one of the best ways of ensuring a fresh, wakeful morning.

Peace

This is one of the most treasured commodities in the world today. Not only do we desire external peace but most of us yearn for internal peace.

The active mind constantly contains meaningless chatter which for some can be quite disturbing. Internal peace can be learned. The chapter on relaxation and meditation in this book can show you how. Some people are extremely fortunate in being able to switch off this nonsensical chatter in their heads. By doing so, they can relax peacefully and switch off from the humdrum of everyday life. This ability is extremely important in the few minutes before retiring to bed at night.

This switch-off comes with the discarding of the day's worries and problems. So, it's not an irresponsible act at all. The unconscious mind continues to work on our problems and their solutions and it does so while we are sleeping. The attainment of this peace of mind before going to bed is probably one of the most important factors in gaining a good quality sleep.

Music and books

I mentioned before that the bedroom should contain a minimum of stimuli to arouse our senses. This includes anything which could remind you of your everyday activities.

The bedroom should be the place to go to switch off. If you do want to read a book or listen to music, that's fine. However, it's important to realise that they should be minimally stimulating and conducive to good relaxation and peace of mind.

Reading something light and fictitious far away from your everyday concerns is more desirable than reading about the world's problems, or economic and financial reports written up in exhaustive detail.

The best form of minimal stimulation before retiring is music designed for relaxing. Many alternative bookshops and some music stores now keep tapes which are specifically designed for relaxing, meditation and reflection. The music is generally soft, slow and of a very gentle nature.

The same tape should be played every night and this becomes a form of trigger or anchor to which our sleep behaviour mechanism becomes accustomed.

All other possible stimuli, particularly those which may come from your spouse, children and friends, should also be kept to a low level. It's a good idea to try to resolve arguments late in the afternoon or early evening so that you don't go to bed with unresolved conflicts that will arise again the next day.

It's a good idea to try to resolve arguments before bedtime so that you don't go to bed with conflicts that will arise again the next day.

Pre-sleep rituals

These are activities normally carried out by people prior to going to bed. For example, brushing your teeth, combing your hair or washing your face. However, there are some things which you can do which will help induce a good night's sleep.

These may include a warm bath or a cup of herbal tea. In fact, probably one of the best ways of ensuring a good night's rest is to sit down quietly and drink a cup of camomile tea or lemon balm tea. If you find these have an unusual taste, then half a teaspoon of honey and half a teaspoon of freshly squeezed lemon juice added to the tea can greatly enhance the flavour.

Certainly a warm bath can also help. In fact, it's recently been scientifically shown to increase the amount of deep sleep. You should avoid hot and spicy foods, sugar, tea, coffee, chocolate and other stimulants as well as alcohol before retiring. In fact, many of these things should be avoided in the afternoon because their carry-over effects can last well into the night.

You should avoid hot and spicy foods, sugar, tea, coffee, chocolate, alcohol and other stimulants before retiring.

Vigorous exercise is helpful for sleep but it should be performed no later than 5 p.m. as it temporarily acts as a form of stimulant. Some light exercise can be performed in the evening about an hour before going to bed, including five minutes of yoga and stretching exercises and a few minutes of deep breathing exercises. This possibly helps to establish a good pattern of breathing during the night and people who practise this report awakening more refreshed.

Massage is extremely relaxing and many people also find that sex is a good way of relieving tension. Meditation and relaxation are also very effective ways of obtaining internal peace and rest (see Chapter 9) — both important prerequisites for high quality sleep. One person who could benefit from this is an elderly woman Elsie, who was reported to me by a colleague.

ELSIE'S STORY

Elsie had suffered from insomnia all her life until she discovered that she was somehow extremely highly positively charged. She discovered that standing on a brass plate in her backyard at night for five minutes in bare feet was sufficient to discharge these positive charges to earth, resulting in an increased feeling of wellbeing and a far better night's sleep.

This is one approach which may be worth trying for those who have difficulty in sleeping and who are responsive to changes in their environment such as humidity, heat, cold and wind changes.

Others who may benefit from this discharging approach are those who feel unwell when they're under powerlines, close to electrical generators, powerful electromagnets and other electrical equipment.

3

Sweet dreams and
BETTER SLEEP FOR CHILDREN

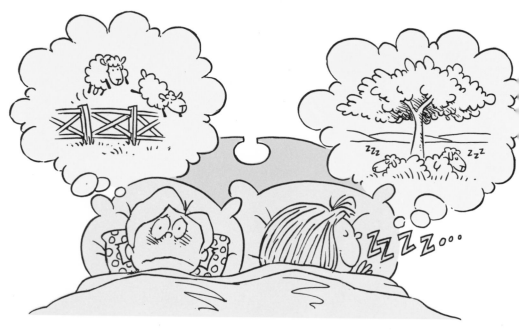

Children may suffer a number of sleep disorders, the main ones being that the child cannot fall asleep, or if the child does fall asleep, then he or she awakens after one to four hours and cannot drift off again.

Sleep therapy, as described later in this chapter, is vital to the management of the sleepless child. Another important consideration is proper sleeping patterns. The child who wanders about the house, crawls into his parent's bed or switches on the TV at full blast in the early hours of the morning, is likely to become an unhappy individual.

Allergies

Stress and psychological factors in a child play an important role but probably dietary factors are the most important of all — they are also often overlooked. The removal of allergenic foods and chemicals after special testing, the use of the tryptophan complex and the love and care of an understanding parent are extremely important. Samantha's story is a good example of how dietary factors should always be suspected in a child's prolonged sleep disorder.

Dietary factors should always be suspected in a child's prolonged sleep disorder.

SAMANTHA'S STORY

Careful clinical investigation showed that Samantha's behaviour deteriorated severely after consuming certain food dyes, particularly yellow and green ones. The behaviour of the seven-year-old girl became so unruly that she became a distraction to the other two children in the family and was the source of most of the disharmony between her parents.

Samantha was diagnosed as being extremely highly sensitive to food colourings to the point that they were acting as poisons. Her family found it difficult to keep her away from these additives, especially when she was at children's parties. On average, these parties would occur once every few weeks and it usually took about four days for the girl to settle down.

At these times, her distractibility in class was pronounced and her attention span and academic performance deteriorated markedly.

One of the most alarming problems was that Samantha didn't sleep at all at night after being exposed to additives and sugar. This affected the entire household. Her parents were rapidly coming to the end of their tether. No amount of psychological support and counselling was of any help.

Finally, it was decided that her mother should educate the other parents holding the birthday parties, and Samantha's teachers, about the effect of colouring on her daughter's behaviour patterns.

Samantha was lucky that the effects of these chemicals on her were immediate and that her mother sought prompt medical help. Unfortunately, some children and adults don't have an immediate and noticeable reaction to these additives and unwittingly expose themselves to low levels for long periods of time. Sleeplessness is a frequent side effect. The end result is often the development of further allergies and illness.

Bedtime rituals

Children's bedtime rituals are very important. This includes going to the toilet, brushing their teeth and combing their hair. Coffee and cola drinks are very damaging to children's sleep patterns and should be avoided.

Very soft music, lullabies or a non-stimulating bedtime story should become an important part of the child's ritual in falling off to sleep. Include a kiss and a cuddle in these pre-sleep rituals. This gives the child the psychological security he or she needs.

Coffee and cola drinks are very damaging to children's sleep patterns and should be avoided.

The bedroom

Make sure that the child's bedroom is warm, comfortable, that the bed isn't too hard, the pillow not too high, that there are no drafts and that it's peaceful and quiet.

For the child who has a genuine need to go to the toilet in the middle of the night, the provision of a small potty beside the bed saves the child a long walk to the toilet or to the parent's bedroom.

Herbal remedies

A small diluted fruit juice with a dozen drops of herbal tincture containing passiflora, ginseng, scullcap, low-dose mistletoe and valerian taken before going to bed can be most effective.

Of course, the dose must be adjusted according to the age of the child and this information is usually given on the label. These herbal drops usually have a very soothing, relaxing and sedating, hypnotic effect on children without becoming harmful, addictive or causing any other side effects.

Herbal drops such as these are known to reduce or stop night terrors, nightmares, sleep walking and moving from bedroom to bedroom, crying, screaming fits and even bed wetting.

Medical causes

If the child or infant is waking at night and appears to be suffering from colic or wind, it's important to look at the child's diet and to remove allergic foods, especially cow's milk.

If the infant is being breast fed, the mother should stop taking cow's milk and replace it with a calcium and vitamin B complex supplement. Cow's milk passes through into the maternal breast milk and can sensitise the child.

The infant or growing child who is not consuming dairy products should receive a supplement of calcium, which will help to induce a very good night's sleep.

Another abdominal complaint which can arouse and awaken the child regularly is the presence of worms. Medical help should be sought for the diagnosis and treatment of suspected worms in the child who can't sleep.

Of course, any underlying medical or psychological causes should be looked for. In particular, low-grade ear, nose and throat infections and respiratory disorders should be sought out and treated.

Sleep therapy

Sleep therapy may consist of a gentle crooning or humming sound or even a gentle stroking of the skin while the infant is asleep.

Sleep therapy has a beneficial influence on the unconscious mind. Animals and the higher apes perform a form of sleep therapy on their sleeping infants. It may be a gentle crooning or humming sound or even a gentle stroking of the skin while the infant is asleep. Instinctively, animals do this for the benefit of their offspring.

Sleep therapy is a very simple and effective form of hypnotherapy. Basically, it's therapy given to the child in the early stages of sleep. The therapy can take the form of requests, or instructions as to how a problem which the child may be experiencing can be solved.

It can be used to help a child with allergies, behaviour disorders, learning problems, inattention, easy distractibility, hyperactivity, sleep walking and especially bed wetting. Nearly every behaviour disorder can be greatly helped by sleep therapy. It's done by giving suggestions to the child within the first forty-five to sixty minutes of his or her falling asleep. The method of performing sleep therapy is simple. When you enter the child's bedroom, after at least forty-five minutes, the bedroom should not be pitch black but should have enough light to let you see movements that may take place in the child during the therapy.

Gently stroke the child's head, repeating in a very soft, slow, gentle voice: 'Stay asleep, stay asleep, stay asleep'. Continue to stroke the child's head and repeat the words until a movement occurs. This may be a movement of the lips, the eyes, a yawn, a lifting of the arms, or movement of the legs.

The child may roll over or even sit up with his or her eyes open, but may still be in a sleep state. Wait until the child lies down again before commencing sleep therapy. No sleep therapy should be given until these movements occur. As soon as movements have appeared, the child will still appear to be asleep. However, this sleep will be light enough for the child to hear but not be awoken by your voice.

Continue repeating softly and slowly: 'Stay asleep, stay asleep'. The unconscious attention of the child will be focusing on your voice and any communication that you make must be carefully and correctly phrased.

Do not use persuasion of any form. For example: 'You'll be happy if I give you some chocolate'. Or 'You will do better in school because I told you so'.

Sleep therapy is speaking to the unconscious area of the mind. It's basically a programming technique. Speak very slowly and quietly with the communication you want to give to the child. Don't whisper. Speak in your normal voice slowly, softly and gently. Repeat the communication five or six times at each sleep therapy session.

Should you have any problem with the form of the communication you should give, or the technique, discuss them with a sympathetic psychologist or psychiatrist. Some professionals are very keen on this method while others have not used it. So, seek out someone who can give you good advice.

If you have any problem with the form of the communication, or the technique, for sleep therapy, discuss them with a sympathetic psychologist or psychiatrist.

The following are suggestions for various problems:
1. You will stop wetting the bed.
2. You will be still and quiet in the classroom.
3. You will no longer need to pick your nose.
4. You will feel happier and happier every day.
5. Every day and in every way you will get better and better.

On completion of this programming, or sleep therapy, the child should be returned to natural sleep by repeating the words: 'Stay asleep, stay asleep, happy dreams, happy dreams, wake up bright and happy in the

Feedback from your child on the communication you're making during sleep therapy is very important.

morning. Mummy (or Daddy) loves you'. Use the child's name where appropriate.

Feedback on the communication you're making is very important. This can be obtained by following this procedure. If you want the child to wake up bright and early, use the following words: 'Wake up bright and happy early in the morning'.

Then, next morning, using the child's name ask : 'Good morning ——, how are you this morning?' The child's reply should be: 'I feel really bright and happy'. Positive feedback from you should occur, but without over-reacting in any way.

Sleep therapy is a dynamic and effective form of help for children. It can be used to suggest that the child will fall asleep as soon as he or she goes to bed. It can also be used to keep the child asleep throughout the night. It can even be used for infants under the age of twelve months with good effects. The key words here are practice and patience.

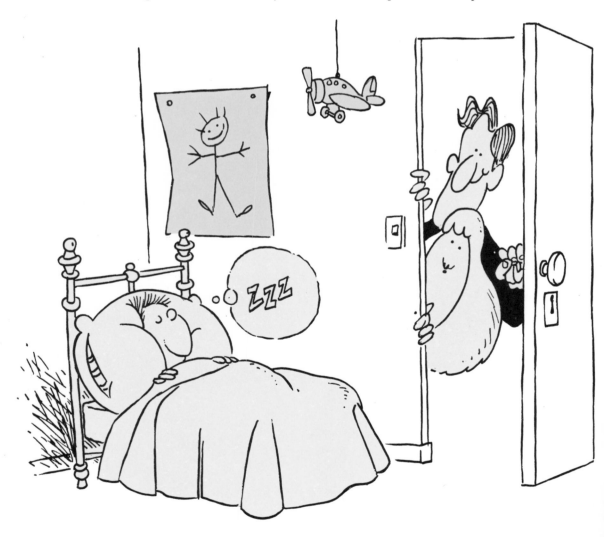

4

Why am I always TIRED?

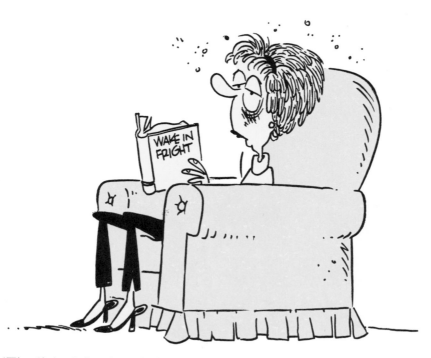

'Tired' is defined as being weary, fatigued, exhausted and no longer willing or able to endure life and its various situations. Fatigue is the diminished ability to carry on our day-to-day work because of a lack of energy. There are many causes of fatigue and tiredness and the causes of these should be eliminated if possible.

An early warning

Daytime fatigue and tiredness is not a normal state to be in, but this problem is very common. Fatigue can be a symptom of the early stages of many diseases, both acute and chronic. It shouldn't be taken lightly.

In fact, many people who develop arthritis, heart disease, and even cancer and diabetes say that they have been feeling tired, lethargic and have lacked energy to do their day-to-day chores for the previous one or two years. Without energy, life becomes dull, boring and eventually depressing.

This lack of energy is not only physical, but it affects the mind and mental functioning as well and can result in loss of concentration, poor memory and such things as 'brain fag'.

Medication

Many of the physical and psychological causes of insomnia are associated with fatigue.

Many of the physical and psychological causes of insomnia (see Chapters 10 and 11) are associated with fatigue and these should be dealt with. Fatigue can also be caused, or aggravated, by many of the drugs which doctors use to treat medical and psychiatric disorders. It's quite possible that the medication you're taking is contributing to, or causing, your tiredness and fatigue. The drugs interfere with the body's state of nutrition and often cause vitamin and mineral deficiencies.

Allergy

One of the most common causes of fatigue and tiredness is allergy. That is an allergy to foods, chemicals, pollution, cosmetics, the water supply and so on. These are important and often neglected causes of many symptoms.

SALLY'S STORY

'I was a real sugarhead. I couldn't get enough of it,' remarked Sally, a thirty-six-year-old working mother who didn't connect her sleep problems with relying on sugar to give her the energy she needed for her busy routine.

'I never felt too good in the morning and usually suffered from a morning hangover, but without the pleasures of the alcohol the night before. My day typically began with a big cup of black coffee with two teaspoons of sugar to kick start me.' Sally's disbelief that sugar could be the culprit, especially in her mood swings, gradually changed over the six weeks it took to wean her off all sugar. Another six weeks elapsed before she felt much better in the mornings and did not crave her sugar fix. She noticed that, at times, she could cause mood swings purposely by eating sugar.

She had no more hangovers or mood swings for the time being. 'But I was still a doubting Thomas. It took me another three weeks to convince myself that this was the cause of my problem. The thing that really made up my mind to avoid sugar binges for life was the tremendous feeling of wellbeing.'

Sally noticed that the severe fatigue she had suffered for a decade, and which would occasionally force her to go to bed for the afternoon, had also disappeared.

Nearly always, allergies are associated with nutritional deficiencies, and low levels of many of the B group vitamins and minerals can contribute to this low-grade chronic fatigue syndrome. The investigation and treatment of these is discussed elsewhere.

Poor quality sleep is another major factor contributing to daytime tiredness and fatigue.

Poor quality sleep is another major factor contributing to daytime tiredness and fatigue. The promotion of good quality sleep is the prime aim of this book. Following the program in the Step-by-step summary of the treatment of insomnia (page 113) should produce high quality sleep.

Here, I would like to discuss three syndromes which are often overlooked and which usually can be easily managed at home. These are the stress-tension-fatigue syndrome, the inactivity-pseudo-hibernation-syndrome, as I have described it, and the post-viral fatigue syndrome.

Stress-tension-fatigue cycle

This particular problem is possibly best described as occurring in an individual who, when in a stressful situation, has learned to become tense and ready for action. The person increases muscle tension in response to a stressful situation and this increased muscle tension results in the contraction of muscles all over the body, including those of the head and neck, the arms, shoulders, back, buttocks and thighs.

If the cause of the stress, be it a difficult work situation or an argumentative spouse, is not removed then the tension in the muscles becomes chronic with the result that the energy reserves in those muscles become depleted. Finally, the muscles become weaker and weaker and the end result is extreme fatigue.

The more fatigue that occurs the less likely the individual is to handle a stressful situation well.

The more fatigue that occurs the less likely the individual is to handle a stressful situation well. The muscles start to tire and weaken even when the muscle energy levels creep up again. These stresses create further tension.

THE STRESS-TENSION-FATIGUE CYCLE

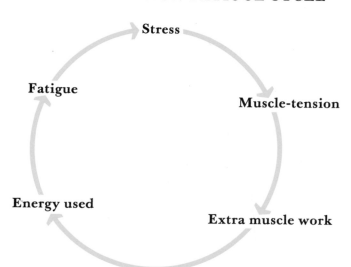

Stress

Fatigue

Muscle-tension

Energy used

Extra muscle work

At any point in the cycle we can do something to break it.

Stress: Relaxation, meditation, lifestyle changes, psychotherapy

Muscle-tension: Stretching, exercise, yoga, tai chi, herbs

Energy lost: Better diet, no refined carbohydrates, vitamins and minerals

Fatigue: Controlled breathing, diet and vitamins, positive outlook, forty winks

This can be a vicious cycle but it can be stopped through retraining. If you have this problem, it's important to attend to the stress reactions and to learn how to handle yourself in situations of stress. It's of some benefit to use affirmations such as 'I'm relaxed and happy at all times', or 'I am totally confident in all situations'. This should be repeated over and over again. This helps the individual to cope well with stressful situations, be they business or social. These affirmations must be practised on a daily basis to become effective.

Another very effective way of breaking the stress-tension-fatigue cycle is to reduce the tension in the muscles. This can be done very effectively using stretching exercises. Stretching exercises are passive in that the muscle groups are stretched one at a time. They are demonstrated on pages 44–47.

If every muscle group in the body is stretched, then the contraction which occurs during the tension cycle is less severe. The muscles are more relaxed and fatigue doesn't set in. Individuals who suffer from the stress-tension-fatigue syndrome quite often feel better after doing a few minutes of light stretching exercises. Fatigue can further be helped by providing the muscles with extra oxygen. This involves slow, deep breathing for ten to twenty inhalations and exhalations.

These simple exercises should be practised on a daily basis. Frequently, the stress-tension-fatigue syndrome can be dramatically reduced or even eliminated completely by performing these simple techniques.

JOHN'S STORY

John was a classic case of job-related stress leading to chronic insomnia. He was convinced that his long-standing problem with insomnia must be because of his sales job. 'It only occurred during week nights. At the weekend and on holidays, I slept like a baby,' said John, forty-six, who finally narrowed the cause of his severe fatigue down to the city air pollution and the air conditioned office he worked in.

He installed an air ioniser in his office on the advice of a friend. This had an almost immediate effect on his fatigue. 'However, as soon as I stepped out of the building, the fatigue would return, as though I were being forced into a heavy overcoat.'

On the days he would come home tired and washed out, he knew he wouldn't be able to get a good night's sleep. Buying a second ioniser changed all of that. Not only did John's sleep improve, but his restlessness and snoring also disappeared — much to his wife's delight.

Activity can help

Although not a syndrome which has been described before, I feel that the individual who is chronically fatigued and can't sleep well may have what I call the inactivity pseudo-hibernation syndrome. I believe that many people who are suffering from chronic tiredness and fatigue, combined with insomnia, are basically people who are inactive most of the time — either they are in sedentary occupations or are invalided and cannot use their body and muscles for physical work.

That describes the inactivity side of it. The pseudo-hibernation part? Well, pseudo-hibernation really indicates that the body and brain have gone into an artificial form of hibernation. The overall metabolism slows down both in the body and in the brain. I believe that these people experience a shut-down in their metabolic activity. The blood-brain barrier no longer allows the transport of nutrients from the blood into the

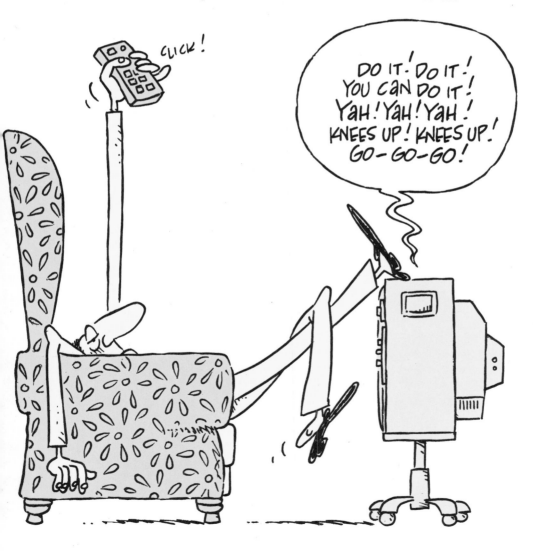

brain as it requires them. Also, the removal of waste products from the brain is slowed down and toxic metabolites are therefore not transferred out of the brain for excretion.

This situation may arise because of nutritional imbalances and deficiencies. More than likely, the presence of chemicals in the environment contributes to this shutting down of the blood-brain barrier. It's probably an adaptive defence mechanism of the central nervous system to prevent it becoming poisoned by environmental chemicals.

The more inactive this group of people become, the slower their metabolic rate becomes. Not only does their physical activity slow down, but also their mental processes as well. The end result is generally gross lethargy, with weight gain and a depressive illness.

The only really effective way out of this situation is to engage in physical activity for at least half-an-hour a day. I have found that within three to six weeks of sustained physical exercise and improved nutrition, this group of people do extremely well.

In fact, many patients who had to take tricyclic anti-depressants or who were given electroconvulsive therapy, probably started as individuals with this disorder. In the early stages of this condition, the sufferer may ask whether sleep is not really the natural state and wakefulness merely a respite for the satisfaction of instinctive drives such as eating and sex.

Certainly, the hibernating individual, or animal, is most unlikely to encounter dangerous predators and stressful situations in the everyday world. Based on this model, the satisfaction of our animal drives would lead to sleep (the normal situation) and their continued frustration would lead to insomnia (the wakeful, unnatural state). For example, if rats are deprived of food they become total insomniacs. The satisfaction of basic instinct and drives generally results in a reduction of activity and drowsiness. This is no better shown than in the soporific effect of the sexual orgasm.

A happy balance in life includes periods of activity and rest — and, on occasions, periods of over-activity and of sleep.

Whatever the situation may be, we must strike a happy balance in life. This includes periods of activity and rest — and, on occasions, periods of over-activity and of sleep.

Post-Viral Fatigue Syndrome (myalgic encephalomyelitis)

The post-viral fatigue syndrome (PVFS) is just another way of describing extreme fatigue following an acute viral illness such as influenza, hepatitis or glandular fever.

The syndrome not only includes severe fatigue, which is the cardinal symptom, but also many other symptoms. Muscle fatigue, especially following minor exertion is the main symptom but muscle aches and pains are also common together with concentration difficulties, short-term memory loss, anxiety, depression, joint pains, headaches, swelling of the glands and intermittent fevers.

The depression associated with this syndrome can be linked to severe insomnia and, at times, over-sleeping at the wrong time of the day. The sleep-wake cycle therefore appears to be interfered with or interrupted in some way.

This syndrome usually affects young adults. However, younger children and older adults can also be affected. The disease itself can cause months to years of severe suffering not only as a result of the extreme muscle fatigue and other symptoms, but also the nausea, indigestion, allergies and the increased risk of infections which follow.

Because doctors often prefer to believe their diagnostic tests rather than their patients, the diagnosis has frequently been missed. In fact, many doctors still believe that the PVFS is 'all in the mind'.

> Many doctors still believe that post-viral fatigue syndrome (PVFS) is 'all in the mind'.

However, the disorder has been described in the British medical literature since the 1930s. The earliest epidemic was in the Royal Free Hospital in London in 1955 when it was called the 'Royal Free disease'. It has also been called the 'Iceland disease', 'epidemic neuromyasthenia', 'myalgic encephalomyelitis', 'chronic fatigue syndrome' and the 'post-viral fatigue syndrome'. It is often inappropriately referred to as 'Yuppie Flu'.

In Australia, more females than males are affected, particularly the young professional groups. It may be that young females seek medical attention for the condition due to sociological factors. Males tend to withdraw if a definite diagnosis is not made, whereas females tend to seek further support and help.

Myalgic encephalomyelitis, PVFS, or by whatever name it's called, isn't a single disease because not all patients have myalgia (muscle pain). As stated, the major symptom is muscle fatigue after minor exertion and this fatigue may be the inability to do anything after getting out of bed in the morning and making breakfast. It may be so severe that simply reading the paper causes gross fatigue in the muscles of the eye, so discouraging the continued effort.

There's also very little evidence of encephalitis in the brain and spinal cord. However, I believe there is an allergic or immunological reaction occurring in the central nervous system which is responsible for causing the headaches and muscle weakness.

The triggering factors differ in different people. Most sufferers can pre-date their symptoms to an acute and severe viral infection. However, others relate the onset of their disease to some bacterial infection involving the use of antibiotics and others even relate the onset of the disease to an acutely stressful period.

It's the responsibility of the individual treating doctor to investigate the background of patients suffering from this syndrome to determine which of these factors was the major contributing cause of their illness.

The germ or virus which actually triggers PVFS in one victim may cause no more than a mild fever in other people. This is fairly strong evidence that the disease has a genetic basis in addition to other predisposing factors. Probably the most important predisposing factor is the state of nutrition at the time of the initial infection, especially in respect to micronutrients and trace minerals.

Persistent symptoms of this disorder actually hint at a profound disturbance of the immune system. The immune system itself doesn't seem to recover from the initial infective insult. Again, I believe this is determined by the state of nutrition of the patient at the time of the initial viral assault on the immune and nervous systems.

It's probable that the organism which triggered the illness results in a severely misdirected immune response. The immune system goes so haywire that it finds it difficult to return to normal activity.

This disease can be extremely crippling. Not only can it cause severe neurological and psychiatric disorders, including insomnia, but being labelled a 'social cripple' or malingerer is devastating. The individual who goes on for years with this problem ends up either divorced, an alcoholic, or a suicide statistic.

According to orthodox medicine, there's no accurate laboratory diagnosis and individuals are usually unresponsive to therapy. However, under the electron microscope, it has been found that ninety per cent of the red blood corpuscles are grossly deformed and lose their normal cylindrical shape. Because the disease is cyclical, often these patients have times when they are feeling quite well. When they are feeling well, the shape of the red blood corpuscles appears normal under the electron microscope. It's also been found that the important helper lymphocytes of the immune system are either low in number or activity in these patients when they feel unwell.

I have found that people with PVFS characteristically have one or more nutritional deficiencies, especially of the B group vitamins, ascorbic acid (vitamin C) and some of the important minerals including zinc. The most effective way of helping these people is through nutritional support including a low stress diet (page 60).

Known 'stress foods' such as white flour, sugar, alcohol, tea, coffee, chocolate, dairy products, chemical additives and yeast should be avoided, and important supplements including vitamin C and the bioflavonoids, B complex vitamins by mouth and by injection, including high doses of vitamin B12 and folic acid, the use of mineral supplements, yoga, oxygen therapies and intravenous vitamin C should be taken.

The very careful use of therapeutic herbs is invaluable in this condition. The important herbs to consider are those which contain high concentrations of bitter principles and cleansing agents.

Early experimental work with intravenous immunoglobulin G hasn't been shown to be of great benefit in the vast majority of patients. However, in a minority of patients it seems to have quite a dramatic effect. Immunoglobulin G is a special solution extracted from human blood which has high levels of antibodies — important factors in fighting infection.

The important thing to remember is that every person with PVFS is an individual with individual requirements and differences.

> **Known 'stress foods' such as white flour, sugar, alcohol, tea, coffee, chocolate, dairy products, chemical additives and yeast should be avoided.**

It's extremely important to remember that prevention is always better than cure. The earlier nutritional therapy is instituted, the better. In fact, at the first sign of an infection, especially a viral infection, it's wise to supplement the diet with the nutrients already mentioned — particularly vitamin C and the bioflavonoids.

Some sufferers of PVFS have found that the bioflavonoids themselves have a mildly stimulating effect which relieves the severe fatigue.

GAIL'S STORY

'Broken and restless sleep during the day does nothing to help my nocturnal insomnia,' was how Gail described the symptom she found most distressing. She had been diagnosed earlier as having PVFS. 'I was an eighteen-year-old schoolgirl then. It wrecked my school year because I was so fatigued that it was a marathon effort to get out of bed and make myself some breakfast, let alone do a full day's study. All this followed a bout of glandular fever when I was sixteen, from which I never fully recovered,' she recalled.

'I felt lethargic, depressed, always tired and had this chronic muscle fatigue. During the day, I only felt I had the energy to move from one chair to another.' Reading was almost impossible as Gail's eye muscles also became very fatigued.

She started taking a low-stress diet, high doses of intravenous vitamin C, intramuscular B complex vitamins, zinc, magnesium and a number of stimulating herbs including ginseng, Gotu kola and cayenne. Within ten days, she began to see light at the end of the tunnel. Some of her symptoms were actually starting to disappear. In two weeks, she no longer needed prolonged afternoon naps and was able to establish a close to normal sleeping pattern. Her energy levels slowly returned so that after moderate activity, her muscles no longer ached and felt like they were collapsing.

Gail was able to do light stretching and yoga exercises which left her with a sense of wellbeing. However, long walks exhausted her and set her back. She found that getting better was a very slow process. 'However, the ability to get back to a full night's sleep and wake up feeling relatively well in the morning has helped a lot,' was how she summarised her progress.

5

Activity helps —
EXERCISE AND SLEEP

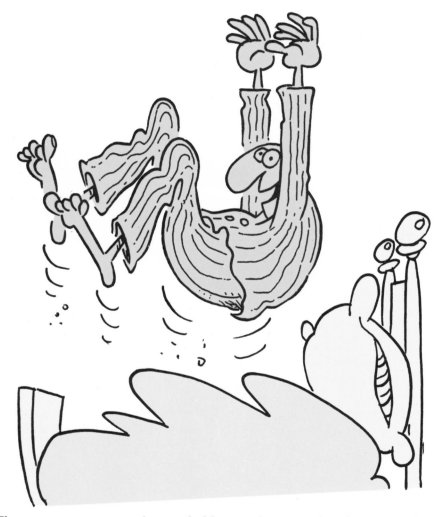

The average person today gets less exercise than any of our ancestors did throughout the history of mankind.

The average person today probably gets less exercise than any of our ancestors did throughout the history of mankind.

With the evolutionary development of our brain and our ability to manipulate our environment, we have developed a string of comforts and labour-saving devices which have taken many of the normal physical efforts out of survival.

We have homes which reduce our needs for finding shelter. We heat these homes artificially which reduces the need for physical effort to produce body heat. We have developed offices and desk jobs. We drive from the comfort of our homes to these desk jobs. The buildings in which we work have lifts, so that we don't have to climb stairs.

We don't even have to move from one office to another to find something out because of the telephone and other communication aids. We don't necessarily have to go shopping either because of the developments of shopping through television and computers.

We don't even have to go out for entertainment because television gives us a prime seat. This reduction in body movement and exercise has resulted in more degenerative disease, less good health and an increase in the rate of psychiatric, psychological and sleep disorders.

Too many of us are flabby and lazy, addicted to convenience foods because it's too much bother to even cook a nutritious meal. Once again, a key point I am reiterating throughout this book is that the body is a marvellous chemical factory as well as a physical machine. Abusing it leads to imbalances, one of which is insomnia. If you look after your body, it will respond in kind.

As I have pointed out before, without adequate and good quality sleep, not only do we suffer from daytime fatigue and lethargy but an increased risk of anxiety, depression, aggression, personality and psychiatric disorders.

Why exercise helps

The maxim: 'If you don't use it, you lose it' rings true. Exercise is very important for everybody. It's important not only to maintain your present degree of health but also to improve upon it in the future. It can also be an effective form of meditation, if you're concentrating solely on your exercise.

Exercise will definitely induce sleep, provided it's done earlier in the day and preferably in the morning if it's extremely strenuous activity.

'If you don't use it, you lose it.'

TREVOR'S STORY

A case in point is Trevor, a forty-five-year-old doctor, who enjoyed participating in marathons as a break from the demands of his medical practice.

Apart from a busy week treating his patients, he managed to run 100 to 150 kilometres a week. During a heavy training period, he noticed that despite feeling pleasantly fatigued after training runs he couldn't sleep. Simply by changing his training time from late evening to early morning, Trevor's sleep patterns quickly returned to normal, despite a period of tiredness in the early afternoon.

This case particularly illustrates the effect exercise can have on sleep if it's done too late in the day.

In the case of people who are ill with some disease, exercise is sometimes quite difficult. I have had patients come to me with virtually no energy with which to exercise at all. They are so run down that even the simplest of everyday tasks such as dressing, walking, shopping and so on are difficult to perform. These activities are also made difficult by painful conditions.

It's therefore very important to start a moderate and graded exercise program daily for short intervals. This exercise should be increased until at least twenty to thirty minutes of moderate exercise is possible.

Improved health and wellbeing

Exercising is useful in improving, arresting and sometimes even reversing a number of serious and debilitating illnesses and diseases.

Exercising is useful in improving, arresting and sometimes even reversing a number of serious and debilitating illnesses and diseases. We certainly know that a moderate amount of exercise can improve our feeling of wellbeing and a certain degree of fatigue and tiredness usually follows exercise.

If we exercise at the appropriate time of the day, with the production of tiredness and fatigue following, then of course we can expect this fatigue will lead us into better sleep. However, it's not only the ability to sleep better which improves with exercise. There are many conditions which have been shown to benefit with increased activity.

LOW BACK PAIN

The best therapy for low back pain is gradual, progressive exercise to stretch the long muscles of the back, buttocks and thighs. There's no better treatment for low back pain than stretching, mobilisation exercises and rhythmical movements to the joints and muscles involved in low back pain.

CIRCULATORY PROBLEMS

Exercise also improves circulatory problems, including those of the heart and the arteries to the legs. The best form of exercise for this is gradual and progressively longer walks. Walking is also an excellent exercise for the back — provided the back is held upright and straight. The muscles are also given exercise during walking.

Lung diseases can certainly be improved with exercise which increases the rate and depth of breathing. For example, tennis, swimming and cycling.

ARTHRITIS

Arthritis also improves with regular exercise, particularly to the joints involved.

I believe that exercise produces substances in the blood which have an influence on the inflammation of arthritis. The body by gentle exercising, can, in effect, produce anti-inflammatory chemicals which dampen down the amount of inflammation present in inflamed arthritic joints.

Therefore, by taking a little exercise, we can avoid taking many drugs.

The old maxim — 'if you don't use it, you will lose it' rings very true in situations of arthritis. I have coined a rather technical term for this called 'panatrophic hypokinesis'. This simply means that all of the organs and tissues of the body become smaller and weaker as a result of a lack of their use.

A classic example of this is a fractured leg in a plaster cast. If the cast is left on for, say, three months, and then removed, the muscles of the leg become much smaller and weaker and they have to be retrained and redeveloped with physiotherapy. Not only do the muscles become small, weak and wasted, but the bones of the leg also become weaker and lose calcium.

ABDOMINAL PROBLEMS

Abdominal and pelvic exercises will help with problems of the stomach, intestines, bladder and sex organs. Exercise benefits people with the irritable bowel syndrome and women with the premenstrual tension syndrome (PMT). It has been found that exercise will even help to relieve the symptoms of allergies, including hay fever, asthma and eczema.

IF YOU SUFFER FROM:

headaches

migraine

insomnia

skin disorders

joint pains or arthritis

abdominal pains and wind

depression

Pre-Menstrual Tension (PMT)

allergies

- **DON'T DRINK MILK**
- **DON'T USE ANY DAIRY PRODUCTS**
unless you can show confidently by tests that they are not harming you.

> Overweight and obese people often have problems with excessive sleep during the night and daytime sleepiness. People in this group may have allergies and nutritional imbalances or deficiencies and should seek medical advice.

APPETITE AND WEIGHT

It is well known that exercise helps to maintain normal weight by burning up carbohydrates and fats.

It is well known that exercise helps to maintain normal weight by burning up carbohydrates and fats. It's less well known that it can help to regulate the appetite. For example, overweight people who sit around all day running an inefficient body system tend to consume more carbohydrate and calorie-rich food than they need. They tend to nibble and snack throughout the day.

On the other hand, people who are active usually eat regular meals at the correct times. The desire for food is usually good but they don't desire more than they need. That is, their appetite regulating mechanisms are very responsive to smaller quantities of food and these mechanisms switch off the appetite for food when sufficient has been eaten. Exercisers are generally not over-zealous eaters.

Exercise has been shown to improve nearly every day-to-day function that we may consider.

Exercise is known to regulate, and reduce, mild to moderately elevated blood pressure. In fact, exercise has been shown to improve nearly every day-to-day function that we may consider.

CONSTIPATION

The lack of exercise and faulty diet contribute equally to constipation. A person who starts a regular exercise program usually finds that their bowels move more regularly and freely with less straining. The bowel actions are usually better formed and easier to pass. Once again, it can be seen that the eliminative process — or the body cleansing processes — are improved by exercise.

Longevity

We have so far been speaking in this chapter about the quality of life and the benefits of exercise. However, what about quantity? When I speak about quantity, I am also speaking about quality.

That is, if we are going to live longer, we also want to live happier, healthier and more productive lives. In parts of the world where we have healthy people living over the age of 100, we know that their activity levels definitely play an important role.

The diets of the longest living people in regions of the world such as the Hunza Valley in northern Pakistan, the Caucasian Mountains of Georgia in the Soviet Union and in Vilcabamba in South America, have diets consisting of living foods that have not been processed.

The foods are usually fresh, seasonal and contain no additives. They have not been put through any process which removes any nutrients whatsoever. In fact, the foods are generally grown 'organically' in rich soils.

These diets certainly contribute to the health and wellbeing of these people, some of whom still bear children when they are over seventy years of age.

These people also lead extremely physically active lives. The Hunzas work steadily in their fields day in, day out. The work is not heavy but it's regular and requires rhythmical muscular movement. They live in valleys and steep mountainous regions which require much climbing. The Georgians in the southern steppes of Russia are also extremely active. Not only do they do physical work but the elderly involve themselves in horse riding and ceremonial dancing at night.

It should be noted that sugar is not consumed in any of these groups where longevity and health are the hallmarks. And, last but not least, they have cultivated good sleep habits to recharge their inner energies.

An exercise program

Starting the exercise program with light stretching type exercise is extremely important. In fact, quite often it's just a few light stretching exercises which will help the body to relax. Even yoga exercises can be of extreme benefit in helping to induce a good night's sleep. We certainly don't want to exhaust anyone with extensive exercise programs to start with. These are not only off-putting but can be damaging.

Good health is largely a matter of careful balance. This is particularly so with exercise and the person who suffers from some sort of disease.

For the relatively healthy individual, gentle, light exercise is the most important to start with. A brisk half-hour walk about one hour before retiring is an excellent way of increasing the body's natural sleep chemicals.

Jogging, swimming and cycling require more exertion and are not recommended prior to going to bed because they do tend to stimulate for a time. This also applies to exercises involving the use of weights, machines, aerobics and vigorous gymnastics.

Whatever exercise is done, it should be enjoyable. Exercise to music is extremely pleasurable and meditative.

Exercise has been shown to be effective in alleviating many disease states and insomnia. It has also been scientifically shown to improve mood, and to reduce depression and anxiety levels over a six-week period. Results are slow but sure.

Whatever exercise you do, enjoy it — and remember, always begin with light stretching exercises to warm up.

BEST EXERCISES

- Walk briskly for half-an-hour each day.
- Plan a physical game with others at least once a week, e.g. tennis, golf, bowling.
- Gardening achieves more than exercise — a pleasant environment and dirty knees gets us back to nature.
- Yoga and tai chi are suitable for all ages.

EACH OF THE FOLLOWING EXERCISES SHOULD BE REPEATED TEN TIMES.

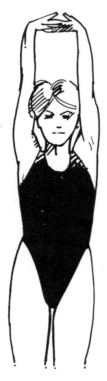

1. SHOULDER GIRDLE STRETCH.
Put fingers together and stretch as high
as you can.

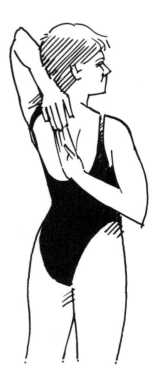

2. SHOULDER GIRDLE STRETCH.
If you can't touch fingers, reach as far
as you can. Repeat other side.

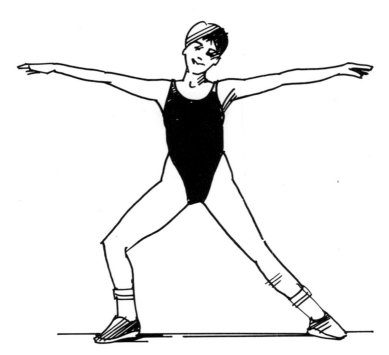

. INNER THIGH STRETCH. Keep body facing front. Repeat with other leg.

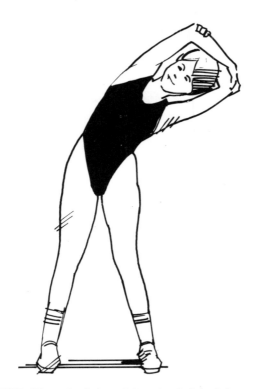

. SIDE STRETCH. Keep body straight, don't bend forward or backward.
Repeat other side.

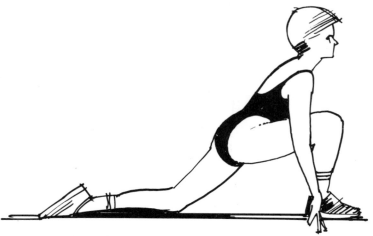

5. HIP FLEX OR STRETCH. Keep knee behind ankle. Repeat with other leg.

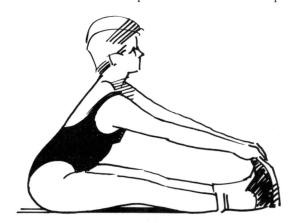

6. HAMSTRING AND LOWER BACK STRETCH. Keep back straight. If you can't touch your toes just go down as far as possible.

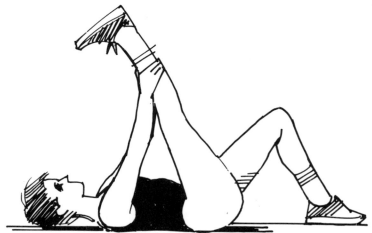

7. HAMSTRING STRETCH. Keep leg straight and knee and foot flexed. Repeat with other leg.

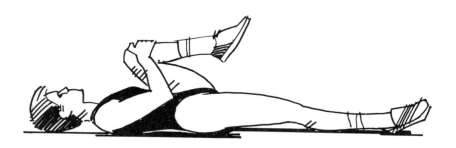

8. LOWER BACK AND LEG STRETCH. Keep lower back and leg on the
ground.

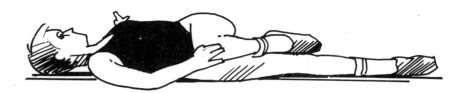

9. LOWER BACK AND HIP STRETCH. Bend knee at 90° angle and pull leg
gently towards ground. Keep shoulders flat on the ground. Repeat with other leg.

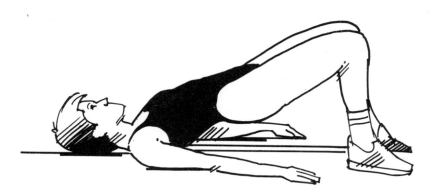

10. BACKSIDE STRETCH. Bend both knees up. Keeping shoulders on ground
and arms straight, lift lower half of torso. Straighten, then slowly lower torso back
onto ground.

6

Food for thought —
DIET AND SLEEP

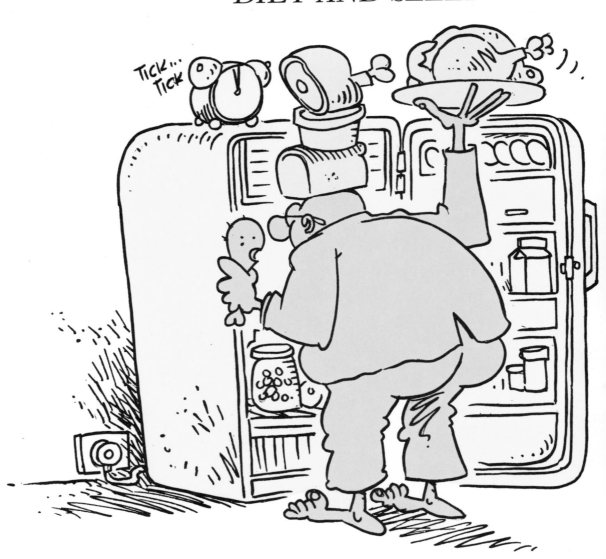

What does my diet have to do with my sleep? It's not always obvious that diet plays a role in sleep. However, it may either help or aggravate your sleep patterns. Your diet contains naturally occurring molecules which the brain uses for its structure and function. Many of these molecules are derived from minerals, vitamins and especially amino acids — the building blocks of protein.

These substances are either directly or indirectly involved in the transmission of messages from one brain cell to another. Some of these messages are stimulating and some are depressing to the nervous system. These molecules which carry the messages are called neurotransmitters.

For example, when we wish to move our hand in a particular way, there are brain cells which release neurotransmitters and send them to other brain cells which control the movement of the hand. The brain depends on our diet for the production of these neurotransmitters. Chemicals in our diet which over-stimulate our central nervous system and brain include tea and coffee, chocolate, sugar and in some cases tobacco.

Substances which depress our central nervous system, or slow it down, include alcohol, sometimes tobacco and many other drugs including drugs such as marijuana and heroin. Carbohydrates and fats also tend to slow down the brain.

Foods may influence sleep patterns in many people in other, more subtle ways. For example, people suffering from food allergies or drug and chemical sensitivities may either suffer from insomnia or hypersomnia. Food additives can stimulate some people.

Others who suffer from reactive hypoglycaemia — a disease caused by consumption of refined carbohydrates, including alcohol and especially sugar — often have anxiety, depression and sleep disorders.

Daily life cycles

Sleeping is an important daily life cycle. Others include hunger and satisfying it with regular meals, periods of activity and rest, and more subtle cycles such as those occurring in the internal organs resulting in the increased activity, or the slowing down, of these organs at different times of the day. It's interesting to note that there are differences in the levels of various nutrients in the bloodstream at different times of the day.

Carbohydrates are better tolerated in the morning than in the afternoon. Amino acids, the basic building blocks of protein, are lowest in the bloodstream between midnight and 2 a.m. Many of these amino acids act as neurotransmitters and this may explain why the central nervous system is at a lower activity level at this time of the night.

Other changes which occur in the bloodstream are variations in the level of cortisone. We know that cortisone can increase the levels of glucose and fatty substances present in the bloodstream.

Changes in the levels of these hormones and dietary substances in the bloodstream have effects on your moods, fatigue levels and sleep. So, it can be seen that the various rhythms which naturally occur in the body happen on a daily basis, are influenced by dietary factors and can have an effect on the quality of sleep.

Sleeping is an important daily life cycle — others include hunger and satisfying it with regular meals, and periods of rest and activity.

The weight factor

Overweight and obese people sleep more than those who are of normal weight. When obese people start to reduce weight, there's usually an associated reduction in the duration of their sleep. The opposite occurs when people who are anorectic start to gain weight. They actually begin to sleep more.

The wrong food at the wrong time

LARGE MEALS BEFORE BED

If you consume an excessively large meal before going to bed, it will interfere with your sleeping mechanisms. A large meal itself requires a lot of energy for its digestion. The absorption of possible stimulating agents in the diet plus the release of hormones in the intestines after the heavy meal can keep you awake for the greater part of the night. It can also alter the quality of the sleep that you have. Some people experience extremely vivid dreams following a heavy meal at bedtime. In some cases, even a small snack can have this effect.

The other detrimental effect of a large heavy meal before retiring is the fact that you are more likely to awaken feeling hung over and heavy.

The best solution is a very light snack of salad as the last meal of the day — and nothing eaten after six or seven o'clock in the evening. A drink of water, vegetable juice or herbal tea for supper is probably the best and safest snack at this time of the day.

In this way, not only are the body and brain given a rest at night, but the gastrointestinal tract is given a rest as well.

EXCESSIVE HUNGER

This can be caused by eating the wrong foods, food allergies, nutritional deficiencies, psychological problems, stress and certain rare diseases of the nervous system. Probably the most common cause of excessive hunger in our community is the consumption of highly refined carbohydrates — sugar, white flour products and alcohol.

Sugar and white flour products are empty calorie foods containing virtually no micronutrients, no vitamins or minerals and very little fibre.

Sugar and white flour products are in abundance on our supermarket shelves. These 'poisons' are empty calorie foods containing virtually no micronutrients, no vitamins or minerals and very little fibre. They are the most highly processed foods available. Rarely are they satisfying in themselves and often the only way of satisfying hunger with these foods is to add fats to them and eat as much as possible.

We see this occurring with fast foods such as hamburgers. They may satisfy the appetite for a short period of time and then on comes the ravenous hunger again. Some people find they become addicted to these foods containing sugars and white flour products and as a consequence they binge on them day in and day out. This maintains their blood sugar levels at a fairly high level throughout the day — but at night, when they're asleep, the level falls to a point where they may awaken in the middle of the night feeling extremely hungry with gripping stomach pains which may even mimic an ulcer.

The first thing that usually happens is the midnight raid on the refrigerator. Usually, they crave something like a carbohydrate meal and get stuck into bread and cheese to satisfy these nocturnal longings.

As mentioned before, these cravings can also be a manifestation of food allergies and food intolerances. People bingeing on dairy foods, tea, coffee, chocolate or even bananas may have an allergy or intolerance to these foods. The foods themselves cause an over, or under, stimulation of their nervous system with a resulting disturbance in their sleep-wake cycle.

Carbohydrates

Carbohydrates contain carbon, hydrogen and oxygen molecules and are present in foods such as potatoes, flour, grains, sugars, alcohol, fruits and so on.

These foods have the most striking effects on sleep patterns. The blood glucose level can be greatly influenced by altering the amount of carbohydrate foods taken at a bedtime meal. A high carbohydrate meal can decrease stage one sleep during the whole of the night and it can increase the amount of rapid eye movement (REM) sleep during the first half of the night. This sort of meal can also decrease stage four sleep throughout the night and it will not only affect the night of the meal but also the following night.

It may be concluded that the relatively high blood glucose levels in people who have a carbohydrate meal at night alters sleep and may lead to a more restful state of sleep. However, this remains controversial because many people experience better sleep without any bedtime snacks whatsoever. It's important to remember that we are individuals and therefore have different requirements.

We know that carbohydrate meals can result in the release of tryptophan which is, in part, converted into a chemical called serotonin in the brain. It is serotonin which is in part responsible for the sleep-wake cycle. In fact, REM sleep is dependent on the level of serotonin — the more serotonin, the more REM sleep is experienced.

Some people who consume large quantities of carbohydrates may feel extremely stimulated during some parts of the day and then all of a sudden drop into a severe state of tiredness and fatigue and have to have a midday or afternoon nap. The consumption of more food then stimulates them into the night and they find it difficult to fall asleep.

Food and chemical sensitivity (allergy)

Foods can produce a wide variety of symptoms in the allergic patient. Chemicals can also produce a vast array of symptoms in most systems of the body.

Not only can food and chemical sensitivities cause eczema, asthma, hay fever, migraines and abdominal pains, but they can also produce subtle changes in the functioning of the nervous system, the immune system and eventually every tissue and organ within the body.

The nervous system is particularly sensitive to food and chemicals. The effects on the nervous system include the aggravation of virtually all psychiatric disorders and psychological symptoms. Symptoms include tension, anxiety, depression, fatigue, mood swings, irritability, weakness, lethargy, crying spells, phobias, irrational fears, visual disturbances, headaches and migraines.

The nervous system is particularly sensitive to foods and chemicals. Problem chemicals can occur naturally in foods as well as in the form of colourings, flavourings, preservatives, emulsifiers and a whole host of other additives.

Chemicals in the environment can also cause problems of a similar nature. These chemicals can occur naturally in foods as well as being added in the form of colourings, flavourings, preservatives, emulsifiers and a whole host of other chemicals which food manufacturers put into our food supply. Chemicals in the air and water can also produce problems. If someone is sensitive to these pollutants, then their nervous system is the system most likely to suffer first. Changes in sleep patterns are very common in people who have food or chemicals intolerances and sensitivities.

It's important to investigate the causes of these sensitivities and to eliminate them from your environment as best you can. Quite often, the food or chemical that you most crave, binge on or find pleasant is the culprit. Those most commonly incriminated are sugars, white flour products, alcohol, tea, coffee, chocolate, cola drinks, all dairy foods (milk, butter, cream, cheese, yoghurt), yeasts and many of the grains.

LINDA'S STORY

Linda, a thirty-five-year-old housewife, had suffered from dermatitis, eczema, mild asthma, a nervous condition and insomnia for many years. She had a craving for milk products and especially certain cheeses. When she gave up eating all the dairy products including cheeses, her asthma disappeared and her skin condition improved dramatically. In fact, only a small area of eczema the size of a dollar coin remained on her arm.

Linda led a very active social life with her husband. She developed a tolerance to cheese and was able to consume small quantities without her asthma and skin flaring up. However, one bothersome problem remained — an occasional night of complete wakefulness. After further talking her problem through, she realised that on the nights when she ate even small morsels of cheese, her nervous system would perk up and remain active throughout the entire night.

Her nervous system was extremely sensitive to cheese whereas her skin and lungs were much more resistant to the effects of dairy products. Unfortunately for Linda, she found that she reacted adversely to even a few crumbs of cheese.

If you suffer from food or chemical sensitivities a low-stress diet is the ideal diet to follow. A low-stress diet consists of plenty of fresh vegetables, fruits, nuts, seeds, brown rice, millet, buck wheat and small quantities of red and white meat including fish. Beverages should include distilled or mineral water, herbal teas and vegetable juices.

If you suffer from food or chemical sensitivities a low-stress diet is the ideal diet to follow (see page 113).

FOOD ADDITIVES AFFECT SLEEP

DEFINITE

Colourings
Flavourings
Preservatives
Sulphites
Monosodium glutamate

PROBABLE

Artificial sweeteners
Pesticide and herbicide residues

WHAT'S LEFT TO EAT?
All organically-grown, fresh, unprocessed ripe foods.

Food additives (especially in children)

Many mothers notice that their children become hyped up and overactive after they have eaten certain foods. Often, they can narrow the cause down to a number of flavourings or colourings in the foods.

It's usually some of the colourings — in particular the red and yellow colourings — which upset many children and over-stimulate them. Once this happens, their behaviour changes and they may become aggressive and quite often uncontrollable.

In the classroom, they become inattentive with short attention spans, and despite often being highly intelligent, they eventually fall into the category 'hyperactive learning disabled'. In the older child, the adolescent and the adult, the socialisation process and higher learning activity in the central nervous system modifies their reaction to these chemicals. Often their symptoms are expressed in other ways including mood disturbances and insomnia. In fact, one patient of mine was a middle-aged man who had never slept for more than one or two hours a night for more than twenty-five years.

Many mothers notice that their children become hyped up and overactive after they have eaten certain foods.

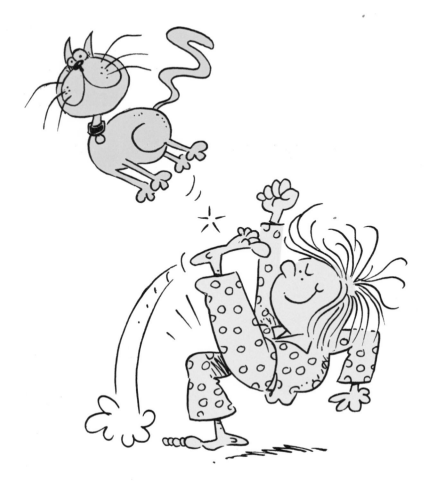

He enjoyed chocolate, other confectionery and soft drinks. The combination of sugar, chocolate, artificial colourings and flavourings was his downfall. However, it was discovered that the major cause of his insomnia was the artificial colourings in the confectionery. It's important to examine the whole range of additives to which an insomniac may be reacting. In fact, it may not be one single additive but a combination of additives which are causing the problems.

Functional reactive hypoglycaemia

Hypoglycaemia is a condition in which the body's blood sugar levels fall below a certain level. This low blood sugar level starves the brain and other body organs of essential fuel.

The brain and central nervous system are very important organs in the body and receive about one quarter of the body's blood supply. They use glucose (blood sugar) and oxygen to produce the energy needed to function.

In hypoglycaemia, there is a lack of this energy and as a consequence the function of the brain and the mind starts to deteriorate. During the day, this can cause a wide variety of symptoms including anxiety, depression, mood swings, fatigue, sleepiness, irritability, heart palpitations, abdominal pains, dizziness, sweating, nervousness and even fainting. Poor concentration and memory disturbances are also frequent.

Of course, if the blood sugar level swings low when the individual is sleeping, then the sleep mechanisms in the brain are disturbed as a result of lack of energy to the cells responsible. The person will then have either a restless night's sleep or will wake up many times during the night.

This problem particularly occurs with people who have cravings for sweets or sugars and who binge on foods containing sugar including cakes, soft drinks, confectionery and chocolates. Often, they don't realise they are bingeing on sugars when they are eating some foods which are highly processed.

It's very important to examine what is present in our foods to determine exactly what types of sugars, and how much, are present. Some of our processed foods may contain up to sixty per cent sugar and we are not aware of it.

A restless night's sleep often occurs with people who have cravings for sweets or sugars or who binge on foods containing sugar.

BLOOD SUGAR LEVELS

Blood sugar

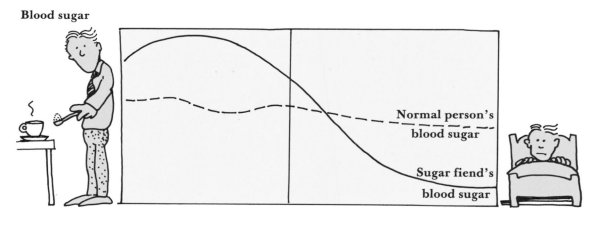

Normal person's blood sugar

Sugar fiend's blood sugar

DAY-TIME   **NIGHT-TIME**

The sugar fiend eats sugar to excess during the day to keep energy levels high. At night the body compensates by lowering the blood sugar to very low levels. This starves the brain of fuel causing insomnia. Raiding the fridge brings up the sugar levels and helps the brain to function again.

If someone is suffering from reactive functional hypoglycaemia, the best thing to do is to completely avoid sugar if possible and to eat frequent snacks of protein-rich foods during the day-time — at least initially. Avoiding all processed foods is critical.

Exercise is also extremely important because it helps control the level of blood sugar. Exercise also evens out the high and low swings of blood sugar and helps to get a good night's sleep. If you have a family history of hypoglycaemia or diabetes it's even more important to take a diet low in refined carbohydrates and have a regular exercise program.

HIDDEN SUGARS

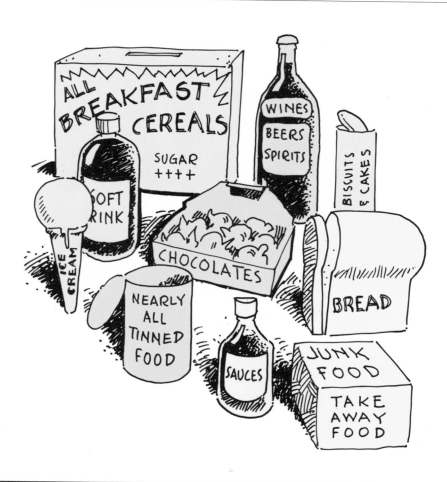

Sugar over-stimulates and over-heats. It's not good for anyone except of course when it's eaten in its only natural state in unprocessed fruit.

Caffeine

Drinks, foods and some medications containing caffeine including tea, coffee, chocolate and cola drinks deserve special attention. Caffeine consumption is probably one of the most common causes of insomnia in the western world today. Caffeinated beverages actually delay the onset of sleep.

Arabian physicians in the eleventh century used coffee to keep sleepy people awake. It was also used back then to keep people awake who took part in marathon religious rituals. The German explorer Reuwolf brought coffee to Europe in the late 1500s and by the early 1600s it had reached England. Its use quickly spread once it was mixed with sugar and made even more exciting and stimulating.

Coffee's addictive nature has been reported in the western world since these early times. The average American consumes approximately eight kilograms of this beverage every year and Australians consume a similar amount. It is, as far as I am concerned, the legalised drugs which cause much harm and ill-health to a large proportion of the population. Not

The average Australian consumes approximately eight kilograms of coffee every year.

JEAN'S STORY

Jean, a twenty-four-year-old secretary for a busy corporation, had slipped into the habit over two years of working sixteen-hour days. 'I seemed to have the office coffee pot continually on the boil. It was a quick pick-me-up whenever I felt low on energy and mentally slowing down,' she explained.

On weekends, she unknowingly developed a craving for coffee. She didn't realise this until it was pointed out by some friends that she was always asking them if they wanted a cup of coffee. Jean realised she had a pattern of headaches developing for twelve months and that these were becoming more frequent and severe. She had resorted to strong painkillers and had consulted a general practitioner and a neurologist to try to find the cause.

She also noticed that she was becoming irritable with people. This contrasted with her previous personality. Luckily, she developed a severe case of influenza. 'I felt like nothing on earth. I didn't want anything to eat or drink — except for fruit juice and water,' she recalled. She was laid up in bed for a week and it took another two weeks for her to fully recover. This flu was a godsend because without it she would have continued to drink large quantities of coffee.

After her illness, she noticed that the first coffee she tried immediately brought on tremors, shaking, headaches and heart palpitations such that she thought she was going to die. When it was explained to her that her allergy had somehow become unmasked by her illness and semi-fasting state, she understood that her coffee addiction, headaches and other symptoms were interrelated. The most remarkable thing about Jean's case is her gratefulness in being able to get a good night's sleep of at least seven hours.

only does caffeine create problems with insomnia, but caffeine-containing beverages may aggravate headaches and migraines, produce pains and spasms in the back, joint and muscle pain, fatigue, over-stimulation, over-excitement and so on.

Every cup of coffee contains about eighty to 120 milligrams of caffeine. Tea contains approximately fifty milligrams of caffeine per cup. Caffeine also occurs in high concentrations in chocolate and cola. It is probably one of the world's most widely-used drugs.

It has been estimated that about one third of individuals in Australia and North America are hooked on caffeine. Caffeine-containing drinks affect different people in different ways. Some people can drink coffee in the evening without it affecting their sleep — or so they think! Caffeine probably interferes with the quality of their sleep but at a level at which they are not completely aware. However, some people assert that even a single cup of caffeine in the late afternoon or early evening will disturb their sleep — sometimes quite dramatically. Why these differences occur isn't clear but some people may be able to clear the caffeine out of their system quite quickly. They are probably those who don't have too many troubles with their sleep.

> **Caffeine consumption is one of the most common causes of insomnia in the western world today. Caffeine is probably one of the world's most widely-used drugs.**

It appears generally that the more caffeine we drink the greater the problem with insomnia. It is recommended that no caffeine-containing beverages be consumed by people who suffer from insomnia — at least not in the early stages of treatment.

Alcohol

Alcohol, as a drug, is also worthy of special mention. Alcohol is not a food. Beverages containing alcohol are not foods either. Alcohol and alcohol-containing beverages are drugs and must be regarded as such. No responsible nutritionist would regard alcohol, and for that matter sugar, as essential nutrients for good health. In fact, the indications are that alcohol and sugar are damaging to the health if consumed even in small quantities over a period of time.

> **Alcohol reduces both the slow-wave, deep sleep and the REM sleep.**

Low doses of alcohol can increase total sleep time and reduce waking activities. The level and the quality of sleep is important. Alcohol reduces both the slow-wave, deep sleep and the REM sleep. These are important phases of sleep and any disturbance to them can only be detrimental. In fact, alcohol can only be regarded as harmful and possibly toxic to the central nervous system. I believe that the effects of alcohol and refined carbohydrates are cumulative and that they may not rear their ugly heads for some years.

> **Alcohol destroys some of the B-group vitamins which are important in normal brain activity and the normal rhythms of the sleep-wake cycle.**

Alcohol is responsible for the destruction of some of the B group vitamins and, as has already been discussed, these are important in normal brain activity and the normal rhythms of the sleep-wake cycle.

Another effect of alcohol is that it stimulates the loss of magnesium in the urine. Magnesium is one of the very important minerals which help to sedate and relax the central nervous system.

So, you can see that there are many reasons for avoiding alcohol at all costs. A little nip before bedtime may help you get off to sleep but it will reduce the quality of your sleep and this will carry over into your next night. Also, with regular use, alcohol tends to cause you to waken after only a few hours' sleep. Thus, short-term sleep gains become long-term health losses.

A little nip before bedtime may help you get off to sleep — but remember, short-term sleep gains become long-term health losses.

Narcolepsy

Narcolepsy is an often overlooked condition. The victim falls asleep at any time during the day without any warning or control. It is not such a rarity in today's high-stress lifestyle with the added complication of a host of food and environmental chemicals to which many people are allergic. Medical authorities don't understand this condition and claim there's no known cause.

BILL'S STORY

Narcolepsy was a dirty ten-letter word to Bill, a sixty-four-year-old commercial analyst. 'My life had been made miserable by it,' he said.

However Bill did have some insight into his condition because his episodes of narcolepsy occurred more frequently during summer months. It was actually after a week of very frequent attacks that his hunch suggested a solution. His wife had noticed him consuming large amounts of tropical fruits including mangoes and pawpaws.

He eliminated all fruit from his diet for four weeks. During this time, his narcolepsy disappeared. On the reintroduction of a number of tropical and stone fruits, it was found that Bill would suddenly, and without warning, drop off into a deep sleep state.

One may tentatively conclude from this, that his narcolepsy was due to a sensitivity of his brain to certain foods. This is what we would call a 'brain allergy'.

Narcolepsy is the reverse of insomnia. However, it can create difficulty in sleeping at night. This case is another example of how foods can influence the nervous system and change its function dramatically.

LOW STRESS DIET

AVOID ALL	DO EAT
Sugar	Fresh fruit and vegetables
White flour products	Brown rice, millet and buckwheat
Alcohol	Wholegrain breads
Tea, coffee	Lean red meat
Cola and soft drinks	White meat
Chocolate	Fish
Tobacco	Nuts and seeds
Illegal drugs	(e.g. pumpkin and sunflower seeds)
Dairy products (if allergic or sensitive)	
Yeast	
Colourings, flavourings, preservatives and other chemical additives	

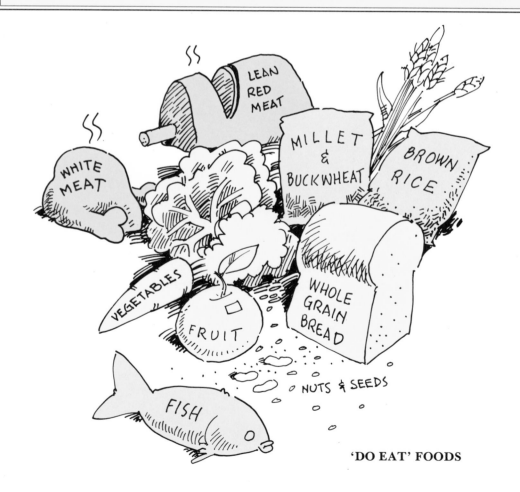

'DO EAT' FOODS

7

The basic building blocks —
VITAMINS, MINERALS AND OTHER NUTRIENTS

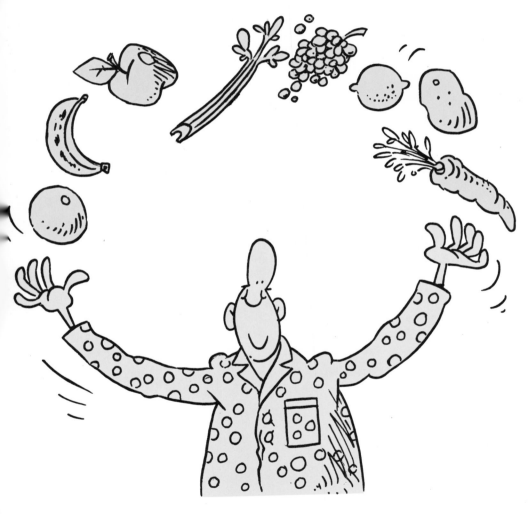

The body, brain and nervous system require basic building blocks for their structures and functions. These basic building blocks come from our diet, water and the air we breathe.

For the body and brain to work best, these building blocks must be supplied in adequate concentration to meet the every day demands and requirements of our system.

KAREN'S STORY

Take the case of Karen. She nominated severe low-energy fatigue and recurring infections as her major problems, pinpointing the time they began as coinciding with the birth of her first child.

A side effect is that I haven't had a good night's sleep since,' said Karen, twenty-three, a part-time secretary. 'I have to keep earning some money as my husband got retrenched from his part-time hotel job'.

Investigation established that Karen's diet consisted of meat, chops, sausages, pasta, eggs and bread. She also drank litres of water a day. Examination of her diet, of course, revealed no fresh fruit or vegetables. She had no taste for these and it was very difficult to convince her to include fresh fruit and vegetables in her diet.

To get the ball rolling, she was prescribed vitamin C with bioflavonoids. These were prescribed in doses of 4000 to 6000 milligrams per day. Virtually the first day she started taking these, her energy levels rapidly returned to normal and in fact she believed they were over-stimulating. Within a week, her insomnia had disappeared and, apart from one or two minor throat infections, that problem also disappeared.

Karen decided that instead of taking pills, she would prefer to eat fresh fruit and vegetables, but she accepted my advice and continued to take 2000 milligrams of vitamin C and the bioflavonoids indefinitely. Karen was very grateful to once more look forward to a sound night's sleep after a demanding day.

Vitamin C is essential for the functioning of every cell in the body — it's as essential as oxygen, water and food. The bioflavonoids improve the action of Vitamin C, especially on the immune system and the brain.

Nutritional deficiencies

Without the basic building blocks from our diet, our bodies cannot function at their best. Our skin breaks down, our lungs become weak and our gastrointestinal tract malfunctions.

If your diet is deficient in protein, carbohydrate, certain fats, vitamins, minerals, amino acids, trace elements etc., the body and mind suffer.

NIACINAMIDE

Niacinamide, or vitamin B3, has been particularly helpful for those people who fall asleep readily but who cannot return to sleep after awakening during the night. The usual dose is between 500 milligrams and 1000 milligrams at bedtime.

Niacinamide has been shown in animal studies to have an effect on the brain very similar to the benzodiazepine drugs. These drugs are the minor tranquillisers which doctors prescribe for anxiety and tension-like states and insomnia.

Niacinamide, in fact, has been found to have anti-conflict, anti-aggressive, muscle-relaxing and hypnotic actions very similar to those of the minor tranquilliser-type drugs.

TRYPTOPHAN

Another very important nutrient for the brain to function is an amino acid called tryptophan. This is a basic building block found in protein. It's converted in the brain to another chemical called serotonin. This is a chemical messenger or neurotransmitter, very important for the induction and maintenance of the sleep state.

The usual dose of tryptophan is approximately one gram taken on an empty stomach forty-five minutes before bedtime. Higher doses may be needed in people over the age of forty who have severe sleep disturbances.

It's wise to take tryptophan with a small dose of vitamin B6 and magnesium because both these nutrients are important for the conversion of tryptophan to serotonin. It's also very important to avoid taking protein before and after tryptophan, as the other amino acids can compete with tryptophan for absorption into the body. However, it's quite safe to take tryptophan with complex carbohydrates.

Tryptophan has been shown in experimental studies with humans to reduce sleep latency — the time taken between lights out and a moderate depth of sleep. Very high doses of tryptophan don't produce any better effect than the moderate doses. In fact, doses above ten grams per day will actually distort sleep rather than help it.

Severe insomniacs who have moderate to severe psychiatric disorders usually don't respond to tryptophan as well. It's possible that their sleep mechanisms have been disturbed by anti-psychotic medications. However, tryptophan and niacinamide are both worth considering for people with severe insomnia. It's imperative to continue treatment for two to three weeks if you fail to respond initially, as quite often, after taking these supplements for some time, an effect will be forthcoming.

The beauty of these forms of treatment is that they have a very low level of side effects when compared with toxic drug therapies. In fact, therapeutic nutrition in general carries with it a negligible number of side effects — and these are usually beneficial, rather than harmful.

If necessary, the dose of tryptophan may be increased from one gram to a maximum of four grams at night. It has been found that tryptophan is also useful for helping infants and children to sleep but the dose must be tailored to their body weight.

The usual dose of tryptophan is five to fifteen milligrams per kilogram of body weight. Infants and children who suffer from insomnia also possibly suffer from food sensitivities — cow's milk is one of the worst offenders.

In children who have insomnia, occasional abdominal pains, diarrhoea

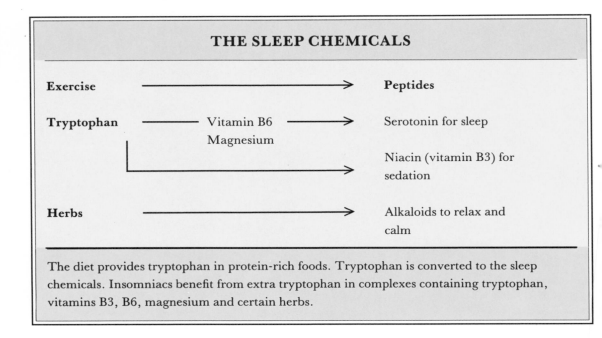

THE SLEEP CHEMICALS

Exercise → Peptides

Tryptophan → Vitamin B6 Magnesium → Serotonin for sleep

→ Niacin (vitamin B3) for sedation

Herbs → Alkaloids to relax and calm

The diet provides tryptophan in protein-rich foods. Tryptophan is converted to the sleep chemicals. Insomniacs benefit from extra tryptophan in complexes containing tryptophan, vitamins B3, B6, magnesium and certain herbs.

and vomiting, always suspect cow's milk allergy. A trial withdrawal may reveal that cow's milk is indeed the major problem.

MINERALS

Other specific nutrient deficiencies have been associated with insomnia. Minerals in this group include deficiencies of calcium, magnesium, potassium and zinc. Low levels of other vitamins can also cause insomnia and these include biotin, folic acid, niacin, pantothenic acid and pyridoxine.

LIONEL'S STORY

A classic example of magnesium deficiency was Lionel, a seventy-year-old retired accountant, who had suffered intermittent cramp and muscle pinching in his legs every night for the past ten years.

Tests confirmed the suspicion that he suffered from low levels of magnesium in his red blood cells. He took supplements of magnesium and calcium and within three weeks his muscle cramps and pinching had diminished to tolerable levels. After six months, the painful symptoms had completely disappeared.

The cramps and pinching prevented him from sleeping but calcium and magnesium are also mildly sedating minerals, which helped improve his sleep.

Choline and inositol are usually associated with the B-complex vitamins but in themselves are not vitamins. They do have some sedating effect on the central nervous system and are worthwhile considering as a useful supplement. Details on the use of all of these supplements can be obtained in the table at the end of this chapter.

EMMA'S STORY

Emma's is a good example of zinc deficiency being associated with insomnia. For two years since she was fourteen, she had been dieting very strictly to control a weight problem and to help with her acne. She swung to an extreme and became totally anorectic. 'I completely stopped eating for long periods of time and lost a total of three and a half stone,' she explained.

For an eight-and-a-half stone girl to lose three and a half stone is horrifyingly dangerous to say the least. Her moods changed and she became very gloomy with a distorted self-perception.

Her mother realised how serious the situation was, and took her to a succession of doctors and psychiatrists, but very little progress was made. When Emma sought help from an alternative medicine practitioner, it was discovered that she had virtually no sense of taste or smell. This is a condition called hypogeusia, which is caused by a zinc deficiency.

This also helped to explain her loss of appetite and the acne and pimples. Some forms of acne are very responsive to supplementation with zinc and vitamin A.

Emma received supplements, both multi-vitamins and minerals and high doses of zinc and although finding it difficult at first, she became less moody and more compliant with the therapy. Essentially, her appetite returned, her moods settled, her acne disappeared and her previously disturbed sleeping patterns returned to normal.

In fact, she found that the dose of zinc, if taken at night, was moderately sedating, and that she had the best night's sleep when taking her forty-five milligram dose of zinc in the evening.

Vitamin C

Vitamin C is relaxing in doses of one level teaspoon of powder and is essential for the treatment of most human ailments.

Vitamin C is essential for most human ailments. It has an effect on the brain by increasing a chemical called cyclic-GMP. This chemical is low in mood disorders. Vitamin C is relaxing in doses of one level teaspoon of powder.

MARY'S STORY

Vitamin C has substantially helped Mary. A forty-seven-year-old housewife, she was crippled with arthritis and looked ten years older than her age. 'I've had precious little sleep in eight years because of rheumatoid arthritis in my neck, fingers, wrists and knees,' she related.

'At times, the attacks would prevent me from having any sleep at all. Without proper sleep, I felt barely alive,' she said, describing how she had only got limited relief from anti-inflammatory drugs and cortisone for most of the eight years.

Mary's doctor prescribed sleeping tablets, but she believed she had become dependent on them. 'They made me depressed and hung over the next morning. I had read a book about curing arthritis with diet and discovered that the avoidance of certain foods, particularly potatoes, tomatoes, capsicum, dairy products, sugar and red meats helped me greatly.'

She also learnt that vitamin C and zinc play a very important role in patients with rheumatoid arthritis. Supplementation with vitamin C and zinc brought further relief over a six-week period. However, Mary still suffered from moderate pains and joint stiffness and immobility. At the end of 1987, she read an article in a women's magazine about the use of evening primrose oil and certain fish oils in the effective treatment of rheumatoid arthritis. She bought a bottle of evening primrose oil.

Within three weeks of taking one gram three times a day, her joint stiffness and pain had completely disappeared. In fact, the swelling and inflammation in her joints also disappeared for the first time in eight years.

Mary looked better, functioned better and decided to take on some part-time work. This involved a substantial amount of walking and bending, which she did with little trouble. She also had no more sleepless nights.

Heavy metals

Not only can deficiencies of certain vitamins and minerals cause insomnia. Excesses of some of the heavy metals can also cause irritability and insomnia as well. Included amongst these are excesses of copper, mercury and arsenic.

Excessive amounts of copper are rare and the most likely source of copper toxicity is drinking water. However, high levels of copper only appear in drinking water which is acidic in nature and which flows through copper piping. The acidic water dissolves the copper from the pipes.

The greatest exposure to mercury comes from mercury amalgam dental fillings, cosmetics, medicines, pesticides and especially seafood and shellfish. Fortunately, mercury can be neutralised in the body by small amounts of the trace mineral selenium.

Arsenic is used in pesticides and may accumulate in workers handling it. Arsenic toxicity ranks second among the heavy metals as a cause of death.

Levels of these heavy metals can be determined by either a blood test, or more accurately, by hair analysis.

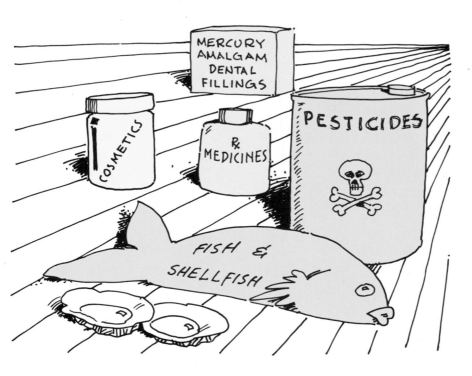

The greatest exposure to mercury comes from amalgam dental fillings, cosmetics, medicines, pesticides and especially seafood and shellfish.

Vitamin B6

Let's end this chapter by giving a case history that many of you can perhaps identify with — the many people suffering insomnia because of a chemical imbalance due to food allergies and a vitamin B6 deficiency state.

JULIA'S STORY

This was the cause identified for Julia's problems. A twenty-nine-year-old mother of two, she described how she had suffered from severe depression and abdominal pains for most of her life.

Her parlous health state, because of food allergies and a vitamin B6 deficiency, had become so serious that she required large doses of vitamin B6 — up to 500 milligrams a day — to keep her depression-free.

Lower doses of vitamin B6 resulted in deficiencies of the vitamin in her blood — Julia had a vitamin B6 dependency state and, at times when her depression became severe, she would increase the doses up to 1000 milligrams a day.

It was also noticed that, at these times, she would have periods of over-stimulation and insomnia. At other times, her whole night would be occupied with vivid dreams which unnerved her. 'My quality of sleep is dreadful,' she complained.

A reduction in vitamin B6 to below 500 milligrams per day resulted in less stimulation and minimal dreaming. Julia is one of those fortunate people whose depression and other problems are easily solved without the use of drugs by changing her diet and giving her a supplement. Her case, however, illustrates that supplementation may cause minor, relatively insignificant side effects which can be quite easily checked by reversing the dose.

VITAMINS, MINERALS AND OTHER NUTRIENTS FOR BETTER SLEEP

NUTRIENT	DEFICIENCY SYMPTOMS	THERAPEUTIC DOSAGE	SIDE EFFECTS OF EXCESS
L Tryptophan	Anxiety, depression, insomnia	½-4 grams (500-4000 mg) an hour before retiring	Unknown
Niacinamide (Vitamin B3)	Fear, worry, depression, headaches, weakness, skin 'burning' sensations, painful mouth and tongue, abdominal bloating and gas, foul abdominal pains, behavioural disturbances, perceptual changes, schizoid personality	100-4000 mg (usually 500–1000 mg per day)	Nausea, itching skin, liver dysfunction
Pyridoxine (Vitamin B6)	Puffiness in face and hands, fluid retention, premenstrual tension syndrome, hysteria, depression, allergies, blank mind, anaemia, dandruff and oily skin, carpel tunnel syndrome, 'arthritis', morning nausea and loss of appetite, cramps and numbness	100-300 mg per day	Nerve damage in doses above those recommended (rare and reversible), vivid dreams, wakefulness, dehydration, loss of short term memory
Calcium	Irritability, tension, grouchiness, depression, muscle cramps, convulsions	1000 mg per day	Calcification e.g. kidneys
Magnesium	Dizziness, heart palpitations, twitching, aching muscles, depression, insomnia, hyper-activity	300-600 mg per day	Drowsiness, sluggishness, coma
Ascorbic Acid (Vitamin C)	Loss of vigour, lassitude, dingy complexion, easy fatigability, lazy, loss of will to do anything, anorexia, fleeting pains in joints and limbs, unwillingness to exercise, sore and bleeding gums, easy bruising, (scurvy and death in later stages)	1000-4000 mg per day (with Bioflavonoids) in divided doses	Loose bowels, wind, abdominal colic
Choline and Inositol	Possible kidney and liver disorders and diabetes	500-1000 mg of each daily	Fishy smell

8

The how and why of HERBS AND SLEEP

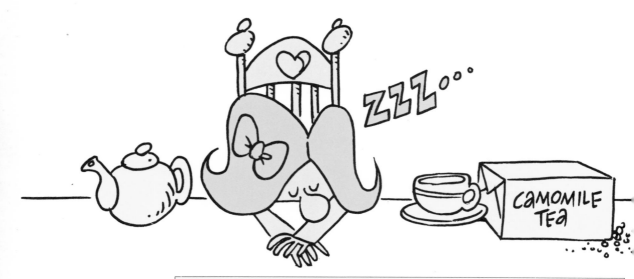

ANDREA'S STORY

Andrea, a thirty-two-year-old divorced mother of four, suffered from severe emotional instability all her life. She suffered extreme mood swings, aggression, temper tantrums, periods of hate, severe depression and frequent suicidal thoughts.

At times of extreme emotional volatility, her insomnia would persists for nights on end. Andrea had tried numerous treatment including drugs, shock treatment, diet, psychotherapy, hypnotherapy, acupuncture, vitamins and minerals and homeopathy.

For people suffering from emotionally attributable disorders with the emotions being the key symptom, the use of Bach flower remedies and herbs is essential. In her case, the Bach flower remedy most applicable was holly. Soon after taking it, her emotions of hatred, anger and jealousy, the very symptoms which had triggered most her other problems, became manageable.

She could now see more clearly why she had reacted in such a way, something which psychotherapy had not achieved although it probably had helped her subconsciously.

Andrea also took a herbal complex containing passion flower, mistletoe, avena sativa, valerian, St John's wort, skullcap and gentian three times a day and at night.

These herbs are essential for the restoration and the relaxation of the nervous system, and in some unknown way, they also alleviate emotional disorders. The herbs must be taken for six weeks to three months in chronic conditions such as this to obtain any lasting improvement. Andrea's case illustrates that one symptom such as insomnia does not usually occur in isolation, but is associated with a number of physical and psychological disorders. Often simple therapies such as these, in the right hands, can produce excellent results, without having to resort to toxic drug therapy.

Some herbs are essential for the restoration and relaxation of the nervous system and can also alleviate emotional stress.

Herbal medicine

In the 1980s, we are witnessing a renaissance of herbal medicine. Despite the great technological advances of organic chemistry and pharmacology, the subtle effects of naturally occurring pharmacological molecules in certain plants has not only great benefit for mankind but causes very little, if any, harm.

Herbal treatments are so old that their misty origins predate humanity. Grazing animals turn to different plants and herbs when they're sick. The world's most sophisticated system of medicine — pharmacology — is being challenged by a system that has been present on earth since animal life began.

Despite the availability of pharmacological drugs developed by our highly inventive and powerful pharmaceutical industry, people of the western world are turning more and more to plants and herbs for treating their illness and the maintenance of their health. Sleep disorders are no exception.

Importantly, these herbs allow individuals to take charge of their own health. They are safer, more accessible and, in the long term, they are more effective than drugs. In fact, even in the orthodox medical literature more publications and articles are appearing on herbs, what they do, how they act and what they contain.

Herbal medicine allows us to take charge of our own health — herbs are safer, more accessible, and in the long term, more effective than drugs.

In fact, a herb called feverfew has recently been given great coverage in the British medical literature for its effect in blocking inflammatory substances in the body. It has been shown to be more effective in treating inflammatory conditions including arthritis, than some of the drugs commonly used.

Evening primrose oil, very helpful for the premenstrual syndrome, is now available under The National Health Service in England for the treatment of eczema.

Most of the valuable drugs we have in modern medicine, including those for pain relief, heart disorders, diabetes and infection (for example, morphine, digitalis, insulin and penicillin) have been derived from naturally occurring substances.

Herbal drugs are safe, effective and available to everyone. However, they are seen as a threat by pharmaceutical companies, which directly, and indirectly, discourage their use. It is indeed unfortunate that some medical authorities in high places seem to be unduly influenced by the powerful multinational pharmaceutical industry.

Anything in excess may be poisonous, including water and oxygen. Yet many seem to be able to justify advocating the banning of a herb or herbal extract because massive doses given to small animals may produce harmful side effects.

Herbs have been used for more than 5000 years in the east by the Chinese. They catalogued and systematised the study and use of plant medicines over 2000 years ago. Herbal medicine and perhaps acupuncture and massage are the only real medicines which have stood the test of time. Synthetic drugs have been with us for only a very short time. Most of them have quickly come into vogue and equally quickly have fallen out of fashion due to side effects.

Nicholas Culpeper, the famous and colourful herbalist of Renaissance England, must be given the credit for making available to the poor of England the herbal knowledge which was jealously guarded at that time by the College of Physicians in London.

These physicians saw the great value of herbs and phytotherapy hidden behind the cloak of the Latin language. Culpeper described the College of Physicians as 'a company of proud, insulting, domineering doctors whose wits were born about 500 years before themselves'.

Culpeper translated all of their valuable information into English and published it for the world to see. He thus put within easy reach of the masses his treatise for effective health care. Consequently, this radical and independent healer was loved by the common people and intensely despised by the surgeons and physicians of that time.

Times haven't changed much. Even the medical profession today may bow to the fact that some of their invaluable medicines are derived from plants — but when one speaks of using pure herbs in medicine the usual response is 'there is not enough evidence'.

The how and why of herbs

It's possible to devise a regime of herbal treatment to help sleep to occur at the desired time which of course should be in the evening. Herbal remedies for insomnia have been used since antiquity — reliably, repeatedly and therefore therapeutically.

It may of course be necessary to prescribe a herb with a relaxing or sedative effect in the evening to help induce a good night's sleep. However, it's equally important to consider the activity level of the individual during the day.

A person who is tired all the time, who has a sedentary occupation, and who lacks physical activity during the day may actually require a restorative type of herb which can generally be given in the morning.

The main aim is to avoid habit-forming drugs and herbs of dependence. It's also important to avoid herbs which have sedative or relaxant effects in patients who have depression.

It's very important to select herbs which have a very gentle activity to start with. These include vervain, lemon balm, lime flowers and camomile. Slightly more sedating herbs which can be used if the more gentle ones fail include valerian, scullcap, hops and passion flower. Only if absolutely necessary should ladies slipper or wild lettuce be considered.

The stronger the herb, the shorter the duration it should be used. Tolerance does develop to some of these herbs and their effect becomes weakened with continued use and without therapeutic necessity.

The stronger the herb, the shorter the duration it should be used.

Before considering the individual herbs used for insomnia, I must emphasise that some of them can be used for other conditions which contribute to the insomnia. For example, a person who suffers from insomnia, asthma and migraine may do better by taking vervain which helps those conditions in addition to insomnia.

Vervain

Vervain, sometimes called verbena, is a herb which acts as a tonic as well as stimulating lactation — the flow of milk from the breast. It will also stimulate sweating.

It's particularly useful for people suffering from nervous exhaustion, asthma and migraine. It has been found to be effective in depression, melancholia, hysterical states, generalised seizures, epileptic fits and gall bladder pain.

Vervain is especially useful in convalescence after fevers, especially those induced by viruses and the flu. The usual dose of the dried herb is two to four grams three times a day.

Lemon balm

Lemon balm, or honey plant, as it's sometimes called, has a mint-like scent. Traditionally, it has been used for anxiety states and to reduce the effects of muscle tension. It has been found to be effective for insomnia in children and because of its pleasant scent, it makes an effective and pleasant drink to be taken after a hectic day.

It also tones up the digestive system and is helpful for people with insomnia, indigestion and other gastric disturbances. The usual dose is two to four grams of the dried herb three times a day.

Camomile flowers

Camomile is a very popular night-time drink in many parts of Europe. There are two forms of camomile — the Roman form and the wild camomile. However, there's not much difference between their effect.

It's the flowers of the camomile plant which are used for relaxing and calming restless individuals with tension. Camomile also affects the digestive system by stimulating digestive secretions. Camomile flowers have mild anti-inflammatory properties and can alleviate some of the symptoms of mild allergies.

Also, in women who suffer from painful periods and insomnia, camomile can be extremely useful. Combined with peppermint oil, camomile helps to relax the large bowel in the irritable bowel syndrome. Individuals with much nervous tension suffering from the irritable bowel syndrome find the combination of these two herbs helpful.

Camomile is especially useful for insomnia in children who are tense and sleepless. Camomile is also an effective remedy for preventing the nausea and vomiting of pregnancy and in some cases it can stimulate the appetite. The usual dose is from the dried flower heads, one to four grams, two to three times a day.

Lime flowers

Lime flowers are especially useful for people who suffer from insomnia and hypertension (high blood pressure). It's a herb which also helps in hysterical conditions, psychosomatic disorders and migraine. The usual dose is two to four grams of the dried flowers three times a day.

Valerian

The herb valerian, also known as 'all heal', is very well known for its tranquilising properties. It also acts as an anti-spasmodic on the bowel, intestines and lungs. It can stimulate the removal of mucous from the chest and it has mild diuretic properties.

Valerian has mild pain-relieving properties as well and may be useful in patients who are suffering from insomnia and painful conditions. It's certainly one of the main choices of herbalists for helping insomniacs and it has definite hypnotic properties.

Valerian's traditional use is for treating severe anxiety states and insomnia, nervous tension and it's certainly a good sedative without the usual habit-forming properties.

It's not depressing in nature when compared with many hypnotic drugs on the market and it does have some minor stimulating properties in that it helps stimulate healing, expectoration and increases the volume of urine produced by the kidneys.

It also helps muscle cramps and tension and can be used for people who have nocturnal cramps. Other uses for valerian include severe hysterical states, over-excitability, hypochondria, people suffering from migraines and also those suffering from rheumatic conditions. The usual dose is one to four grams of the dried root three times a day.

Scullcap

Scullcap is also known as helmet flower and mad dog weed. It relaxes the central nervous system and it has very good over all healing properties as well as being an effective anti-spasmodic.

It's particularly useful in people with insomnia who have epilepsy, including Grand Mal epilepsy. It can improve general health and slow the disease process in some patients who have multiple sclerosis and other neurological disorders.

The nervous exhaustion and debility following acute viral infections also responds to the use of scullcap. The usual dosage is a half to two grams of the dried herb three times per day.

Hops

Hops is the herb used in the production of beer. Its actions include a general antiseptic and sedative effect. It's particularly useful for insomnia, neuralgia (nerve pains, especially in the face), nervous tension, indigestion and mucous colitis.

It's not wise to use hops if you suffer from depression because the hops can aggravate depressive illnesses. The usual dose is a half to one gram three times per day.

Passion flower

Also known as maypop, or grenadille, passion flower is the flower which produces the well known passion fruit. Its specific use in herbal medicine is as a hypnotic herb for the treatment of insomnia. However, it's also of benefit to people suffering from heart palpitations, asthma, nerve pains or neuralgia and, in some cases, Grand Mal epilepsy.

Passion flower does have some pain-relieving properties also and, if used over a period of time with other herbs, has been found to be extremely healing. The usual dose is a half to one gram of the dried plant three times a day.

Herbs that nourish

There are certain herbs which can actually restore the diseased nervous system to normal, or near-normal function, by providing nourishment in the way of specific substances.

They are basically nourishing herbs and don't act either as stimulants or relaxants to the nervous system. By restoring its molecular status, an over-excited or depressed, under-active nervous system will return to normal.

These herbs are usually used over long periods of time in such conditions as shingles, neuralgia and degenerative conditions of the nervous system including multiple sclerosis. Even severe psychosis may respond with prolonged use of some of the restorative herbs for the nervous system.

Persistence must be applied to their use. We are talking about the use of these herbs for two to six months and waiting patiently for the response.

The most common herbs used are common oats, damiana, St John's wort, vervain, squaw vine, rosemary, Gotu kola and Asian ginseng.

It may be found that some of these herbs are either mildly stimulating or relaxing in their own right. They must be used with care. Ginseng and Gotu kola are also known as adaptogenic herbs. These are herbs which help maintain normal functioning in the face of acute or chronic stress.

Some herbs actually help to restore the diseased nervous system by providing special nourishment.

In effect, these herbs help to modify the body's stress reaction. The end result of this, of course, is to allow the body to cope with stress and prevent it from breaking down with the consequent development of degenerative disease.

Be prudent when selecting some of these more widely acting herbs. Although not always necessary, it can be of benefit to have the opinion of a qualified medical herbalist. For example, something totally outside the nervous system may be influencing an individual's inability to sleep.

Again, insomnia, mental depression and intellectual sluggishness may be the result of poor circulation which may be helped with circulatory stimulants such as horseradish, ginger or cayenne.

You can see that the prescription of herbal remedies is sometimes simple, but it can also be a complex matter which is best handled by the professional herbalist.

Herbal preparations

It's generally best to use herbs in their fresh form — either as tea or as an infusion.

Herbs of course are a natural part of the environment. However, many medicinal plants are not available in the cities and areas where people live and sometimes have to be imported

It's generally best to use the fresh plant — either as a tea or as an infusion. If the fresh plant isn't available then we have to resort to either specially prepared fluid extracts and tinctures or dried herbs in tablet and capsule form.

In fact, if the dried herbs in tablet and capsule form are taken with plenty of fluid, they are generally as effective as the other forms.

Herbal extracts are easier to give to infants and children. Often, the herb can be given in the child's fruit or vegetable juice, or it may be given in a little glycerine or pure honey.

The herbs must be taken as directed on the bottle or as prescribed by the medical herbalist because these substances do have medicinal properties and an overdose can produce side effects.

It's important to use reputable brands of herbal preparations whether they be tinctures or tablets because the better companies preparing these medicines put the raw herbs they are using through strict quality controls. They select herbs which have been properly grown in the right environment and under the right climatic conditions. They insist on the herbs being harvested at the time when the active ingredients are in maximum concentration.

Storage and handling of the herbs are also important factors in the eventual effectiveness of the herb, because many volatile compounds can be lost through evaporation if kept at the wrong temperature.

SEDATIVE HERBS	STIMULANT HERBS	NUTRIENT HERBS
Vervain	Horseradish	Common oats
Lemon balm	Ginger	Damiana
Lime flowers	Cayenne	St Johns wort
Camomile		Vervain
Valerian		Squaw vine
Scullcap		Rosemary
Hops		Gotu kola
Passion flower		Asian ginseng
Ladies slipper		
Wild lettuce		

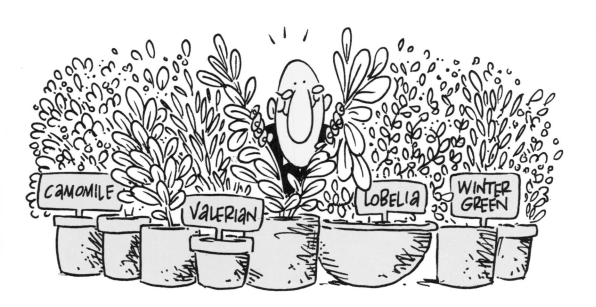

9

We all need to relax —
RELAXATION AND
MEDITATION

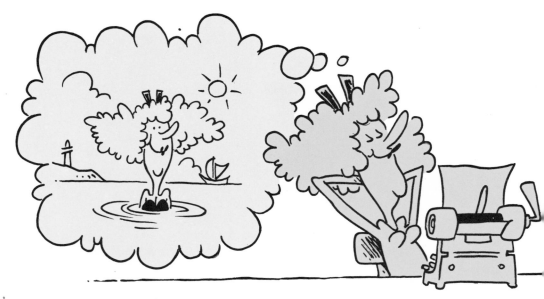

Relaxation

We all need to relax our mind and body at least once a day. In some societies, it becomes almost a ritual to relax once, twice or more often throughout a busy working day. For example, some Middle-Eastern and Eastern religions require their devotees to stop their day-to-day routine and bow to Mecca or pray to God frequently. Even the non-religious Yogis of the East suggest punctuating the day with periods of rest and relaxation.

Everyone, no matter what their age or occupation, needs to have rest. The daily cycles of life and living dictate that periods of rest and activity are normal and that they are in-built mechanisms in every living thing.

Remember, just a few minutes relaxation at the same time every day is probably worth more to you than all of the hustling and bustling of everyday life. Relaxation isn't harmful. Drug therapies often are. Complete relaxation and rest from your daily routine will bring renewed vigor, energy and peace of mind to the rest of your busy day. The question is — how do we do it?

Relaxation is an art and it's one of the aspects of daily living that is not adequately taught in schools or to our children generally. As babies we had developed the art of relaxing and switching off. As we become exposed to more external pressures and stimuli, these detract from this natural process of 'shifting into neutral gear'.

One of the best definitions of relaxation is to rest and enjoy yourself. To me, this means to stop doing and thinking about your everyday cares and worries and to turn away from the routine external environment. The idea is to focus on your pleasant thoughts — whatever they may be. Focusing on a different and pleasant activity is another way.

At the beginning, this requires a certain amount of training and discipline to actually be able to concentrate on past experiences which have been of immense pleasure. It can also be concentrating on planning future similar experiences.

The ability to concentrate within yourself is a learned activity. It requires practice and patience. It's simple and easy. One of the most effective ways I have found to achieve this centering ability is to concentrate on your breathing. There are many different techniques for learning how to breath for relaxation and meditation and the following is probably as good as any.

One of the best definitions of relaxation is to rest and enjoy yourself. Focus on your pleasant thoughts — whatever they may be.

BREATHING TO RELAX

Remember the last time you were tense and upset about something? What happens to your breathing? With most people under situations of tension, stress and anxiety, their breathing becomes more rapid and shallow. This short, rapid breathing actually promotes more tension and anxiety.

The Ancients knew that the control of breathing can control other activities in the nervous system. By reducing the rate of breathing, that is, by increasing the depth and time between each breath, it's been shown that not only can the breathing be slowed down but the rest of the activity in the nervous system also slows down.

This results in a feeling of relaxation. Thus, it can be seen that breathing rhythms and cycles are linked with the state of activity of the brain and mind. When you're calm, you breathe slowly and regularly. But, when you're tense and anxious, you breathe quickly and shallowly. By controlling the breathing, and therefore the brain and mind, we can switch off this tension.

One of the simplest, most effective ways of controlling breathing is the following exercise. Sit on the floor with your legs crossed and your back straight. Concentrate on breathing out slowly through your nose. As you breathe, imagine a feather being held a few inches away from your nostrils.

Concentrate on breathing in, and breathing out slowly through the nose so that the imagined feather hardly moves. The slower and the deeper you can make the breaths, the better. At the beginning, this may seem difficult, but concentrate on it.

Count the number of seconds it takes to inhale and exhale each time. When you start these exercises, you may only be able to breathe in to

In situations of stress and anxiety our breathing tends to become more rapid and shallow — when we are calm and relaxed we breathe slowly and regularly.

the count of five seconds and out to the count of five seconds. Practise increasing the number to ten seconds on inhalation, and ten seconds on exhalation.

When you have achieved this slow, rhythmical breathing, you can increase the counts up to twenty seconds. Count slowly and quietly to yourself. In time, you will be able to make this practice a routine with which you can punctuate your day. You may find that doing it once or twice a day is sufficient to keep you relaxed. You may even find that by performing these controlled breathing exercises four to six times during the day, you feel better, have more energy, work more efficiently and have greater control and intuition.

Once you have learned to control your breathing like this, a short period of controlled breathing exercises before retiring is an ideal way of slowing down your breathing rhythms and activity in the brain.

With slow, gentle, rhythmic, controlled breathing, all mind and body activities follow naturally.

Don't worry about any other fancy techniques of breathing because, once you have mastered this technique, you're well on the way to self-control and relaxation. Remember, the feather in front of the nose. It should still be there and slightly quivering towards the nose on inhalation with a very gentle movement away from the nose on exhalation.

This is how slow, deliberate and gentle the breathing should be. This is what life should be. With slow, gentle, rhythmic, controlled breathing, all mind and body activities follow naturally.

CONTROLLED BREATHING

Practise three times a day
Practise when feeling early stress
Remember:
    longer breaths
    slower breaths
    deeper breaths
Practise before bed

Meditation

Meditation is probably the single most powerful therapy in the management of any disease. It has been practised for centuries in eastern countries to maintain health and wellbeing and to aid in recovery from illness.

Meditation provides one of the most basic ingredients of good health. Its psychological effects include relief from tension and anxiety, and a feeling of inner calmness. The physical effects include the relief of pain and physical discomfort, the reduction of metabolic activity, the activation of the immune system and the normalisation of many physiological activities including heart rate, blood pressure and respiration.

Meditation creates a definite mental harmony and emotional balance in people who practise it. Coinciding with this improved mental harmony is the improvement in overall wellness and the ability to sleep better.

WHEN THE APPLE IS RIPE

'When the apple is ripe it will drop from the tree of its own weight.' This Eastern proverb beautifully sums up the meaning of meditation. The meditative process acts as a catalyst to organise the body's chemistry into a whole. The mind has profound influences on your degree of health. Even in sickness it can play a role either by improving the degree of wellness or worsening the degree of illness.

Not only do thoughts and emotions influence your behaviour, but these very thoughts and emotions can play a direct role in influencing all of the body's subtle physical and chemical actions and reactions.

The time-honoured method of meditation has recently become very fashionable in the management of many illnesses, including cancer, AIDS, psychosomatic disorders, pain and high blood pressure. Not only has it become popular, but it has been scientifically validated as a method of improving physical and psychological functioning. A spin-off of all this improvement of course is more energy during the day and better sleep at night.

A POSITIVE APPROACH

The act of meditation generates positive behaviour and attitudes without effort or cost. With a modest investment of time, meditation can take you to a higher plane of wellbeing and a totally different perspective on your existence.

Meditation is the foundation for optimum health. It is not a religion but a way of life. Meditation is concentration within. It is effortless. It's just as if you're falling down a well within yourself. Others have described it as a 'diving within'.

Meditation is simply the process of being able to effortlessly let go of everything while concentrating on one thought, one word or one idea. In fact, simply sitting and knitting can be regarded as a form of meditation. By passively sitting in a chair in a slightly uncomfortable position

Practised for centuries in the East to maintain health and wellbeing, meditation is probably the single most powerful therapy in the management of any disease.

'When the apple is ripe it will drop from the tree of its own weight.'

with your eyes closed for twenty minutes twice a day, you can eventually achieve a state of relaxation or meditation.

The mind is allowed to wander and invading thoughts are allowed to pass through consciousness. Eventually the concentration within starts to dominate. This may take days, weeks or months depending on the individual. All thoughts are eventually blocked out using this process.

By achieving the ability to switch off in such a way, this well-practised habit of meditation can be applied in the evening before bedtime. By allowing the mind to calm itself, sleep naturally follows. The intellect is gradually phased out. It's not necessary to think during the meditative process. No conscious effort is required and increased feelings of inner peace, deep relaxation and serenity usually develop. Eventually, even the feelings of inner peace fade away to be replaced by a state of selflessness. This gently progresses into a deep feeling of unity, or oneness, with the entire self and your surroundings.

When you are at peace with yourself, not only do you feel better within but you can notice improvements in your relationships with those surrounding you.

TIME AND PATIENCE

The 'meditation habit' takes time. It cannot be developed overnight or even within days or weeks. A slow transition occurs in yourself after you have practised meditation for several months. This change is slow but sure. On a day-to-day basis, changes are usually not very noticeable. However, over several weeks blending into months, you will find tremendous changes.

'Do not push the river.' Meditation proceeds at its own speed and reaches its goal in its own time.

Meditation proceeds at its own speed and reaches its goal in its own time. The whole process should be allowed to flow naturally and slowly. It has what the Zen Buddhists have when they say: 'Do not push the river'. In other words, don't try too hard.

INSOMNIA AND OTHER DISORDERS

As mentioned before, meditation can help a large number of disease states which may, or may not, be associated with insomnia. It has helped dozens of my cancer patients and hundreds of my patients with immune disorders and allergies.

People who meditate say that they can cope better with the realities of life. They become more resilient to external, irritating factors and they feel more together 'within' themselves. They have more energy, feel more spontaneous and less tense.

It appears that their whole coping and adaptive mechanism improves. Over all, people become more cheerful and optimistic and find that they can more easily accept their day-to-day problems. However, there's a cost — time and self-discipline.

It's equally important for a person who is well as it is for someone suffering from cancer, AIDS or some other severe disease to approach meditation with a deep degree of sincerity, openness and a genuine desire to learn about themselves In other words, it's a feeling of needing and wanting to reach out for something deeper and more meaningful.

I know of people who have undertaken meditation and have found that previous experiences can be relived extremely vividly. They note that their reactions to these experiences in the past may have been inappropriate and immature. By reliving these experiences and by changing their responses purposefully, a sense of greater self-esteem and personal growth results.

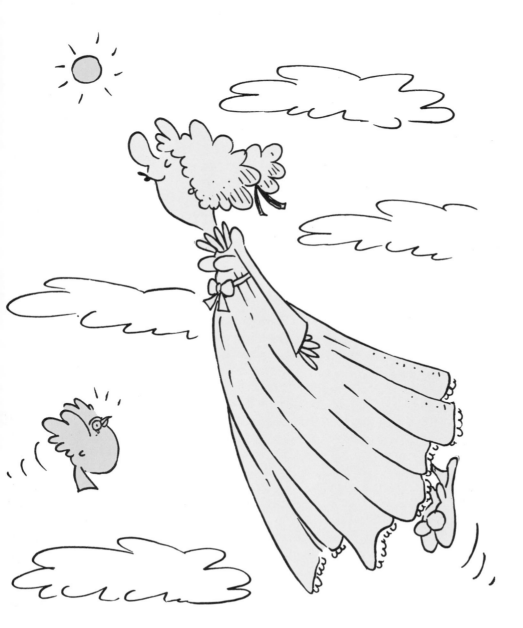

SIMPLE, NATURAL, EFFECTIVE

Meditation is a simple therapy. It can be practised at any time. In fact, the Japanese in their crowded trains travelling to and from work are often practising their meditation. They are not asleep and inattentive as it might appear. Rather, they are actively concentrating on their relaxation and meditation.

It's safe and sure and a method which can be used by all including children. Meditation is not prayer and it's not a religion. It's not self-hypnosis but it does resemble such a state of mind. It's also not a form of magic or a secret formula derived from ancient mystics. The state of meditation is certainly not learning the ability to develop alpha brain waves or any other fancy scientific explanation.

Meditation is a natural process. Observe your pet dog or cat lying in front of a warm fire. They're not always asleep when their eyes are closed. In fact, your pet is probably meditating on the soft warmth of the fire and the homely sound of voices.

Meditation is a natural activity and may be as simple as sitting knitting or listening to music with your eyes closed.

As I mentioned before, meditation is purely natural and it may be as simple as sitting knitting, sitting listening to music with the eyes closed, or more seriously, the purposeful sitting in the lotus position with the eyes closed concentrating on a word or thought.

Meditation is not a form of psychotherapy, although many people find it psychologically helpful. Meditation is simply a state of being and knowing within. The practised meditator will discover what this eventually means. The key word is practice.

PRACTISING EFFECTIVE MEDITATION

The successful practice of meditation requires a little time and self-discipline. With this investment, however, you will find that your life can be dramatically changed. Not only will insomnia, minor aches and pains, frustrations, anxieties, tensions and problems seem much better but the risk of developing serious illness is greatly reduced.

However the determination to meditate must come from within yourself. For someone suffering from insomnia, and the disorders associated with insomnia, this is often quite difficult at the beginning. The discipline needed to spend half-an-hour twice a day on meditative practice must come from a genuine desire within for self-improvement.

Two half-hour daily sessions are recommended for a reasonably healthy individual. Some of my very sick patients, those with cancer and AIDS, who are benefiting from diet and meditation spend two to six hours a day meditating and claim great improvement. Their secret is self-discipline and if you are willing to apply it, there's no reason why you can't beat your insomnia and the symptoms which go along with it.

Select a quiet room and use the same place each time for your meditation. The bedroom is ideal. Lock the door and either take the telephone off the hook or turn the bell down. Make sure that you're not distracted by anyone or anything, including distracting thoughts.

The room must be very, very quiet. It's important to select the same time every day to meditate. That is, it's very important to develop a good meditation habit. Choose a chair which isn't too comfortable. A comfortable chair will enable you to fall asleep. The best chair is one in which you're sitting without back support.

The best time to meditate is early in the morning and late in the afternoon. You must meditate twice a day. Each time you meditate, you should take twenty to thirty minutes — therefore you will be meditating for forty to sixty minutes daily to start with.

When you do become more familiar with the routine, you will naturally increase your meditation time if and when required. It's possible to meditate for six or more hours a day. This may be necessary for some very sick people. However, my recommendations are forty to sixty minutes daily for most people. Once in the habit of meditation, a ten-minute session in the middle of the day can be quite relieving and invigorating.

You must carefully prepare yourself for each meditation session. Don't use alcohol or stimulants such as tea, coffee, tobacco, or other drugs before meditation. In fact, it's not really a good idea to use these at any time. It's also important not to get excited or involved in an over-stimulating session with friends or workmates.

It's better to meditate before a meal than after. Experienced meditators find that an empty stomach is more conducive to the true meditative process. If you need to attend the toilet, then do so. There's no point in meditating with a bowel or bladder that's wanting to empty itself. Be as comfortable as possible. Wear loose clothing but sufficient to keep you warm in the winter. Sit perfectly quietly on the edge of your chosen chair, straighten the back and hold your head up. Attempt to emphasise the curves in your lower back as much as possible. Your hands should be placed on your lap close to the knees. At this stage, you're ready to allow your thoughts to flow freely 'like a river' while concentrating on your breathing. The concentration on the breathing should be on definite, slow inhalations and exhalations. Imagine a feather in front of the nose just moving towards and away from your nose with each inhalation and exhalation.

A state of free thinking is the key to successful meditation. Don't worry about pleasant, or unpleasant, thoughts appearing. In time, your thoughts will change in a way that will help you to meditate more effectively. In fact, if you're in the habit of choosing two or three short affirmations, then repeat these over and over again at the beginning of each meditation session. In this way, your thoughts can be concentrated on to a few affirmative sentences.

Affirmations which are ideal to start with are: 'I feel good about myself.'; 'Every day, in every way, I'm getting better and better.'; 'I'm relaxed and happy at all times.' You can, of course, make up your own.

Meditation is easy, simple and it works — but remember, you should meditate twice a day in the same place for at least twenty to thirty minutes.

Don't use alcohol or stimulants such as tea, coffee, tobacco or other drugs before meditation.

JUST RELAX AND LET IT HAPPEN

Breathe very slowly inwardly and outwardly through your nose. It's possible to reduce the amount of breathing to two or three breaths or less in a minute. Don't force yourself at all. I repeat, the entire process is meant to be effortless.

It's easy, it's simple and it works. But, remember — twice a day in the same place for at least twenty to thirty minutes. Don't expect immediate results or rewards. These come in time. Make meditation a lifetime practice and many of your problems will be solved — and the others will seem less important.

BEFORE MEALTIMES IS BEST

It's recommended that meditation be done before meals rather than afterwards. Mornings and late afternoons are when most benefit can be derived from the meditation sessions. The effects of meditation are not conducive to immediate sleep despite its calming and restful effects.

The effect on sleep and insomnia come as a result of the altered state of physiology of the body and mind. That is, if we can remain relaxed calm and peaceful during the day from our meditation sessions, then the fall of night comes with a feeling of peaceful fatigue and the desire for natural sleep.

Excessive food can influence sleep and disturb our state of rest. It can also disturb our ability to meditate and focus on a particular thought. It's unwise to eat immediately before or after a meditation session because food itself can interrupt the delicate and subtle physiological changes which occur.

From this form of meditation, you will only gain what you are prepared to give. Once you have become an experienced meditator you will get more from the meditation than you actually put into it. Most people find that it usually takes from one to three months before they know if they're benefiting from the sessions.

Again, this depends on the individual and the amount of time you have devoted to the discipline of the meditative exercise.

AWARENESS AND ENERGY IMPROVE

A change in your level of awareness is probably the first change which occurs in the first few months of meditation. Sometimes, this occurs earlier and, within a period of days to weeks, meditation brings results. Also, by being able to relax and switch off the stresses and tension during the day, the stress-tension-fatigue cycle can be interrupted.

Meditation is a form of recharging your batteries. However, the increased level of relaxation and the reduction in anxiety levels are two of the more obvious changes which occur in the early phases of the meditative process.

It's important to realise that meditation is a total clearing of all thoughts and fears. Invading thoughts are allowed to enter and become a part of the mind for the process of meditation. However, attempts should always be made to clear these thoughts as soon as possible.

Repetition of affirmations is one way of switching off thoughts which may appear to be too intrusive. Of course, fears and guilts will arise as will past experiences. These must also be dealt with in the same way. Not by blocking them off but by allowing them to flow freely.

If they become persistent and over-invasive, then attempt to waylay them by using your affirmations. Allow thoughts to enter the mind and to pass through unhindered. This constant practice will allow you to gain control of your thoughts, actions and behaviour and, indirectly, it will result in you being able to control your insomnia.

KEEP THE MIND AS A FORM OF REGISTER

You must attempt to treat the mind as a form of register. The register must be cleared at the beginning of each session. Alternatively, it can be thought of as a tape which can be magnetically cleared of all information at will. When the tape is replayed, nothing appears on it.

This is what's meant by the process of meditation. The mind should eventually be clear of all thoughts. In time, an experienced meditator can apply meditation anywhere — in a busy train, at work, or on the top of a mountain. However, to start with it's desirable to meditate in a comfortable, quiet, familiar place. As I have mentioned before, the bedroom is ideal. Don't worry if the whole process seems slow. It is! Things are still happening to you but at a pace at which your mind and body will allow. The important points to remember are regular practice and don't try too hard.

COOKING A SMALL FISH

The two most common mistakes are trying too hard — and not trying enough. Trying too hard happens when you try to concentrate too much or begin to intellectualise or become impatient and attempt to speed up the whole meditative process.

On the other hand, not trying enough occurs when you slip out of your routine of meditating twice a day. Don't let the sessions become superficial by allowing distractions to occur.

Also, insufficient attempts at meditation occur when you cut the session short or fall asleep. The Chinese describe this process of doing but not overdoing as like 'cooking a small fish — you must be careful not to overdo it'.

WITHOUT EFFORT

The experience of meditation will take you into a realm of quiet and subdued expectancy in which you become open and receptive to everything.

This is an effortless process requiring time and self-discipline only. Experienced meditators become attuned to everything. But, they hear or see nothing at first and have no expectations of what is to occur before,

The two most common mistakes when you begin to meditate are trying too hard — and not trying enough. As the Chinese say, it's like 'cooking a small fish — you must be careful not to overdo it.'

or after, the meditation. They are therefore really never disappointed.

Whatever happens to them is usually for the best. As far as you are concerned, the meditation process requires virtually no effort at all. However, the rewards of meditation come when you are ready. They come at their own speed, and in their own time, and they cannot be hurried.

The rewards certainly won't come on demand. With patience and persistence however, many people, whether they have cancer, arthritis, AIDS, painful conditions or simply irritability, anxiety, depression and insomnia, can benefit from this simple and easy process.

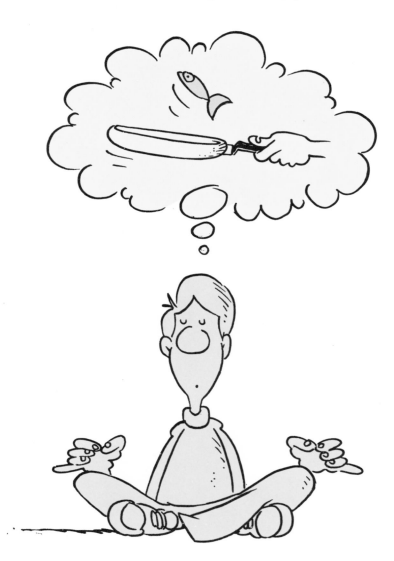

10

The medical causes of
INSOMNIA

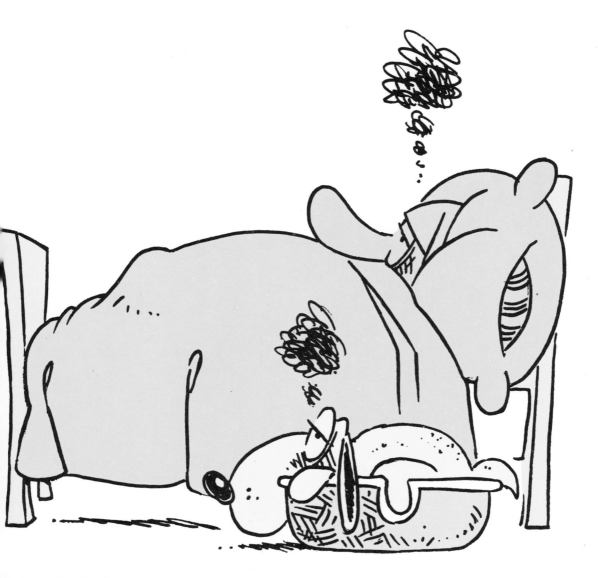

Pain is the single most common medical cause of insomnia. This pain may result from a range of common, and not so common, diseases. An underlying factor in many such causes is allergy.

Insomnia respects no age or rank. Take the case of ten-year-old Frank.

FRANK'S STORY

As well as insomnia, Frank suffered the symptoms of hay fever and nasal stuffiness which had troubled him for the past five years. He also had learning difficulties at school with consequent behavioural problems. His mother was concerned that his hay fever might develop into something more severe such as asthma and this, rather than the insomnia, was why she sought treatment for him from a medical practitioner practising herbal medicine.

Frank was found to have food and inhalant allergies, including allergies to dust and house dust mites. When his diet was changed and his inhalant allergies were treated with desensitisation, his teacher noticed an almost immediate improvement in his behaviour and school work. He was no longer listless and lethargic in the classroom but was a happy, bright, alert boy. His nasal stuffiness and hay fever disappeared. However, possibly the most dramatic improvement his mother noticed was a full and restful night's sleep.

As well as food and inhalant allergies, people may suffer chemical allergies.

ARTHUR'S STORY

Tryptophan is very helpful for insomnia related to chemical sensitivity problems. Such a case was Arthur, a fifty-six-year-old carpenter who for many years had been treated for a moderate anxiety and depression state with tranquilliser and anti-depressant drugs. Because he was convinced that his symptoms were due to some physical components in his environment, he was tested for allergies. The allergy investigation showed he was allergic to the fumes from glues he had been using. He was also found to be sensitive to a number of other chemicals and to one or two foods.

Fortunately, Arthur was in a position where he could change jobs in the building firm so that he wasn't exposed to the fumes. He was treated with dietary supplements and massive doses of intravenous vitamin C. During this time, it was found that his drug medication could be slowly reduced until he was totally free of them.

In the last few weeks of drug withdrawal, Arthur began experiencing extremely vivid dreams and fantasies which disturbed him. It was concluded that this was probably due to the high dose of vitamin B6 he was taking. This was reduced and his dreams became less troublesome. The supplementation with tryptophan finally stopped these annoying side effects of drug withdrawal. 'I now feel the best I have in thirty years,' was his parting comment.

Asthmatics really know what insomnia means night after night.

JILLIAN'S STORY

Jillian, a thirty-three-year-old housewife, had suffered from asthma since the age of sixteen. 'I knew I was in for a sleepless night whenever the coughing, shortness of breath and wheezing came on,' she said. 'Even with the asthma under control, I discovered I was having increasingly more sleepless nights.'

On questioning her, it was discovered that her asthma inhalant contained a drug which, while causing the airways to open up, was also causing her to have a tremor in her hands. Jillian's asthma and insomnia disappeared when her diet was changed and she took supplemental vitamins and herbs specific for her condition. The conclusion here was that the drug used to treat the asthma was actually causing side effects including the tremor, shakes and unwanted brain stimulation.

Of course, not every asthmatic can stop taking medication as Jillian did. The fact that all drugs have some side effects is often overlooked and medication changes may be needed in people who suffer side effects.

Activity also plays a very important role in ensuring a good night's sleep. Many medical conditions cause people to reduce their activity. This leads to a vicious cycle where lack of activity causes sleep disturbance and lack of sleep causes reduced activity and so it goes on.

MOLLY'S STORY

Molly, an active volunteer working for several charities, was increasingly finding that her ability to do anything had deteriorated markedly. 'I blamed this on my inability to sleep,' explained Molly, a fifty-five-year-old diabetic housewife. 'I had been using insulin for about fifteen years and believed that my diabetes was under control.'

This was confirmed by blood tests. However, there were times when her blood sugar levels did go a little high. It was found that Molly's only abnormality was a low level of zinc, vitamin E, vitamin C and chromium in her system. She was given supplements of these and her blood sugar level stabilised extremely well. In fact, she was able to slowly wean herself off insulin.

Molly noticed an increase in her energy levels to the point where she returned to almost full-time voluntary work. Only after an increase in her activity levels did she start to have a good night's sleep with a healthy dream recall. She has now become a crusader for natural medicine and healing.

Painful or discomforting disorders

> ### TONY'S STORY
>
> Tony's problems began when a crane prematurely released a load of bricks he was guiding by hand on the construction site where he was working as a labourer. He suffered severe muscle, bone and joint damage to his upper and lower back, legs and arms.
>
> Tony was initially treated with painkillers and physiotherapy. However, this gave him little relief. His pains became increasingly worse and more generalised so that his whole body ached for most of the time. This resulted in severe psychological depression and, of course, insomnia.
>
> 'I'm only thirty-three and want to get back to work,' he said with frustration when he first came to see me. He was taken off all high-stress foods and was placed on a nutrient supplementation program with some improvement. At this time, he also began acupuncture treatment which gave him some temporary pain relief.
>
> Tony's depression, pain and insomnia continued despite the use of large doses of all of the appropriate vitamins, minerals and herbs. It was finally decided that he should take D-L-phenylalanine — an amino acid important in preventing the breakdown of the body's own pain-killing substances called endorphins.
>
> This isn't in itself a painkiller but a very slow-acting brain chemical which increases a person's pain threshold. After four weeks, Tony's pain and depression had markedly improved and his insomnia disappeared. Three months into the treatment, a formerly very sick and unemployable building worker had become remarkably well and was looking for work.

Pain is the most common symptom for which patients seek medical help. Pain can best be described as a very unpleasant experience, usually associated with some sort of tissue injury, damage or disease.

Pain is a sensation perceived as varying degrees of discomfort, sometimes to the point of being totally intolerable. This is one of the sensations from which we desire to have immediate relief. Pain is very rarely regarded as a pleasurable experience. When it is, it should be regarded as being part of a psychiatric disorder.

There are many diseases and conditions associated with pain, including arthritis, irritable bowel syndrome, migraine and headache, sinusitis, low-back pain, period pain and so on. These conditions should be treated individually, either medically or by some alternative such as transcutaneous nerve stimulation (TENS), acupuncture, chiropractic manipulation or herbal medicine.

Pain can be aggravated or even caused by certain foods in the diet. The anti-stress program outlined at the back of this book will often help to alleviate the pain. Surprisingly, coffee is a substance which can promote pain. There are chemicals present in coffee which block the effect of the brain's own naturally occurring painkillers — the endorphins. It's not just the caffeine in the coffee which does this. There are other preparations present in instant coffee which can promote pain. They stop the brain's naturally occurring pain-controlling opiates — the endorphins — from effectively operating. Therefore, pain will be felt unnecessarily.

Enkephalins are substances produced by brain cells to stop pain. Enkephalins are produced in the presence of copper. The production of enkephalins is reduced if a person is copper-deficient, either by not consuming adequate copper in the diet or by using large quantities of zinc and iron as supplements.

Probably the most important nutrient substance in the relief of pain is a substance called D-L-phenylalanine. This is an amino acid which occurs in the diet and which stops the breakdown of enkephalins in the central nervous system. When the breakdown of enkephalins is stopped, we have an increased amount of them in the central nervous system. Therefore we tend to feel less pain.

Supplementation of the diet with D-L-phenylalanine may be helpful in people who have suffered with chronic pain — even when standard medication and painkillers have provided limited or no relief. The dosage of D-L-phenylalanine is 750 milligrams half-an-hour before meals daily.

At least three weeks' treatment must be carried out before its effectiveness can be ascertained. After three weeks, if there hasn't been any relief of pain, then the dosage should be doubled for another three weeks until a response is obtained. Unfortunately, D-L-phenylalanine doesn't work with everyone. However, it's worth a trial when painful conditions have been persistent. It's also useful in some cases of depression. D-L-phenylalanine shouldn't be taken by anyone suffering from the uncommon disease phenylketonuria.

Again, tryptophan is useful in chronic pain. The usual dose is two to four grams daily and it must be taken away from meals, especially protein-rich meals. Pain tolerance has been shown to increase in patients with severe facial pain, dental pain, headaches, postoperative pain and also low-back pain. It must be remembered that tryptophan should be taken with a small dose of vitamin B6 and magnesium to allow it to become effective.

The following herbs are also of use in painful conditions. We have already mentioned valerian. This is good for the nervous system generally, and for tension and anxiety states. It can also be used for chronic pain but does take some time to have an effect.

Wintergreen is another herb which is effective in pain relief, especially for rheumatic and arthritic conditions and muscle disorders.

Lobelia is a herb restricted to use by qualified practitioners. Lobelia is also known as Indian tobacco and is very effective in asthma, bronchitis and some nervous disorders.

There are chemicals present in coffee which block the effect of the brain's own naturally occurring painkillers — the endorphins.

The underlying cause for the pain must always be treated. A careful, clinical search must be made by a qualified medical practitioner to find out why the pain exists. However, pain may be present without serious underlying disease. It's for these pains that natural treatments are most effective. As I have previously outlined, these treatments include mineral salts, vitamins, amino acids, herbs, homeopathic remedies, acupuncture and chiropractic manipulations.

Generally, they're not toxic and are inexpensive ways of dealing with one of mankind's most common ailments — pain. The effective management of pain can result in not only a greater sense of wellbeing but also in better sleep.

The effective management of pain can result in not only a greater sense of wellbeing but also in better sleep.

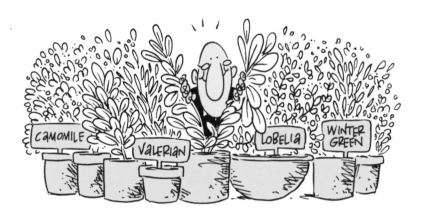

Cramps

Cramping in the legs, especially the calf muscles, is common in elderly people with arteriosclerosis. It may also occur in athletes and people who use their legs a lot. These cramps often occur at night in bed and can be quite severe, painful and persistent.

The best way to manage this problem is to take adequate amounts of calcium and magnesium salts, building up the dosage until the cramps subside. Potassium salts are also of benefit.

A good, high-potency multi-mineral preparation available in health food stores and pharmacies can often do the trick. It may require one or two weeks of supplementation, increasing the dose on a weekly basis, until a positive response is obtained. The uptake of the calcium can be helped by supplementing the diet with some cod liver or halibut liver oil capsules which contain vitamin D. This helps the calcium to be absorbed into the system and better utilised. Interestingly, vitamin D also appears to have cancer-protecting properties.

Arthritis

There are many forms of arthritis but the most common is the 'wear and tear' form — osteoarthritis. The best treatment for any arthritic condition is to evaluate any foods or chemicals which may be aggravating the condition, removing all offending foods and last, but not least, exercise frequently as though your life depends upon it.

The evaluation of vitamin and mineral deficiencies and imbalances, and the provision of nutrients which help alleviate the condition, is essential to build up the tissues around the bones and joints. One of the best vitamins for this is niacinamide, or vitamin B3, which has been discussed in the section on anxiety. For people who suffer from both arthritis and insomnia, the most effective nutrient supplement to date is evening primrose oil. This contains an essential fatty acid known as GLA which is used by the joints to reduce inflammation and swelling. Consequently, there's a reduction of pain and an increased ability to move the joints and perform work.

The other effect of this nutrient, GLA, is to travel to the brain cells and improve their function. By doing so, it generally makes people feel more energetic and relaxed when they take a supplement of evening primrose oil. It's particularly beneficial for lower back pain and spondylitis associated with the premenstrual tension syndrome.

Evening primrose oil usually comes in 500 milligram capsules, and the dose is one to two capsules three times a day. Vitamin C, with the bioflavonoids, in doses of between 4000 to 8000 milligrams per day, is also very useful for arthritis. Vitamin C also has some minor tranquillising and anti-depressant properties. If there's an allergic component to the arthritis and insomnia, then the use of calcium ascorbate can be particularly useful. A level teaspoon of calcium ascorbate powder in juice twice a day 'keeps the doctor away'.

A herb which is particularly useful in the treatment of arthritis and which also has some pain-relieving and sedative properties is devil's claw. It's useful for treating generalised rheumatism, arthritis, gout, muscle pains, lumbago and some forms of tenosynovitis and fibrositis.

Another important aspect of arthritis is that many people become inactive because of joint pain. This inactivity is the worst thing for both the arthritis and the insomnia. If you suffer from arthritis you should exercise to the limit of your ability. This of course should not be taken to painful extremes. Swimming is an excellent form of exercise for arthritics as are yoga and tai chi. The more exercise a person with arthritis gets, the better their general condition, their arthritis and their insomnia because all three are linked.

> The more exercise a person with arthritis gets, the better their general condition, their arthritis and their insomnia — because all three are linked.

The premenstrual tension syndrome (PMT)

This is the collection of symptoms which occurs in females in the week or ten days before the onset of their period. During this time, there's an increase in anxiety, tension states, depression, spontaneous weepiness, physical symptoms such as swelling of the breasts, abdominal bloating, headaches, loss of sexual appetite and frequently quite severe mood swings and changes in personality.

This is thought to be due to an imbalance in the female hormones at that time of the month. However, there are many dietary factors which play a role in women who suffer from the premenstrual syndrome and these include an excessively high intake of salt, refined carbohydrates such as sugar, white flour and alcohol, caffeine, dairy foods and yeast.

Again, the low stress diet (page 60) is ideal because it provides many of the B group vitamins and minerals which women need at this time of the month.

Probably the most useful nutritional supplement for women with PMT is evening primrose oil in doses of 500 to 1000 milligrams three times a day. Taken over a period of two months, most women usually find that primrose oil, B group vitamins, magnesium, zinc and in some cases even vitamin E, can be of great benefit.

Acupuncture can be quite effective, especially points around the inside of the lower legs where they are tender, just above the ankle. You can massage these points yourself twice daily to obtain relief.

Exercise helps women with the premenstrual syndrome but, as we

Acupuncture can be very effective in treating the collection of symptoms associated with premenstrual tension.

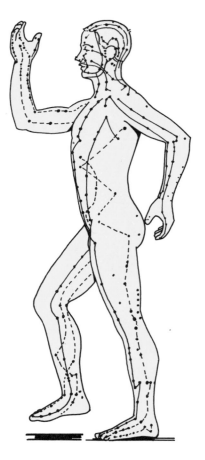

This acupuncture chart shows the courses of some of the 59 meridians that direct the body's flow of vital energy.

have mentioned, the evening primrose oil seems to have the best effect over all, including its ability to induce a good night's sleep.

Infections

Recurring infections of the ear, nose and throat or chest, especially in children, can result in quite a disturbed pattern of sleep. Some children suffer from up to eight or, in some cases, even ten bouts of infections to the lower or upper airway every winter. They receive course after course of antibiotics with no real reason being given as to why they are getting these infections. The simple fact is that their immune system is under stress from foods or chemicals. It's also crying out for nutrients like zinc and vitamin C. Simply, by removing some of the stress foods, especially sugar and dairy products, their infections often settle down and sometimes completely disappear.

> **Recurring infections of the ear, nose and throat or chest, especially in children, can result in a disturbed pattern of sleep.**

Many of these people will respond to supplementation of vitamin C, bioflavonoids, zinc, cod liver oil, a small dose of vitamin B complex and a dose of garlic. These nutrients either boost the immune system or help to suppress the growth and development of bacteria, fungi and viruses in the system.

A dose of zinc at night time in children who suffer from recurrent infections is often sufficient to sedate them and so give them a reasonable night's sleep. So zinc is actually performing a number of functions. It's not only important for the health of the immune system, but is also imperative for the wellbeing of the emotional centres in the central nervous system and the brain. Certain herbs including camomile and lemon balm, discussed in the herbal section of this book, are particularly useful for children.

Sleep apnoea

This is a syndrome which may be due to partial obstruction of the upper airway during sleep. It's characterised by a loud snoring followed by periods when the sufferer temporarily stops breathing. As a result, low levels of oxygen occur in the blood often to quite dangerous and life-threatening levels. Symptoms associated with sleep apnoea include severe tiredness during the day, a deterioration of intellectual capacity, changes in personality, impotency, morning headaches and abnormal movements during sleep.

It's believed that the obstruction in the airways occurs in the voice box, or larynx where the vocal cords are. It's suggested that there's a spasm of the vocal cords which results in this condition. It's more common in obese men, and often their wives quite descriptively diagnose the condition.

Children with large or infected tonsils also often suffer from sleep apnoea with daytime tiredness, irritability and behaviour and learning disorders at school. It can also result in strain to the right side of the heart.

Other people with sleep apnoea, who are often overweight, also complain of only falling asleep several times a week. They can be labelled 'hyposomniacs'. The only thing which may help them is a general improvement in lifestyle, including increasing daytime activity, exercise, diet changes to reduce weight and the use of anti-stress supplements (see summary on page 113)

An element of allergy may be contributing to the spasm of the vocal cords. If you suffer from sleep apnoea, and especially if you have any other symptoms of allergy including skin rashes, migraine headaches, arthritis, irritable bowel syndrome or a past history of asthma, eczema or hay fever, it would be worthwhile having yourself tested for allergies.

The avoidance of any drugs or herbs with sedating effects would be wise. However, vitamins, minerals and tryptophan could certainly be helpful. Ginseng, cayenne and Gotu kola are non-habit-forming 'stimulating' herbs worthy of a trial for this condition.

High blood pressure (hypertension)

This is a common disorder in our society. In most people, the cause is unknown although dietary factors probably play a significant role in the development of this symptom.

We know that high salt and alcohol consumption contribute to the development of hypertension. In some people, food and chemical sensitivities will also increase their blood pressure.

Emotional stress produces elevated blood pressure. Deficiencies of calcium, magnesium and some of the B vitamins may also allow the blood pressure to rise. The deficiencies aggravate emotional stress. A high fibre diet, or preferably a vegetarian diet, will help to lower the blood pressure in a large number of people. Of course, the avoidance of caffeine, alcohol and salt and more exercise will also contribute to significant blood pressure reduction.

Food and chemical sensitivities are probably the main reasons for most hypertension. Sugar has been shown to produce an elevated blood pressure in both animal and human studies. The investigation of these sensitivities is imperative in anyone with hypertension. The possibility of lead or cadmium toxicity is also an important factor and can be determined by a hair analysis for these heavy metals. A hair analysis consists of the collection of a tablespoon of hair from the nape of the neck. This hair is then analysed for lead, cadmium, arsenic, mercury and aluminium.

Drugs used in the management of high blood pressure can often cause anxiety and depression — for example, beta blockers can cause restless sleep and nightmares.

Drugs used in the management of high blood pressure can often cause anxiety, but more particularly depression and impotence in men. The drugs may also have an adverse influence on sleep patterns. For example, beta blockers can cause restless sleep and nightmares. Therefore, investigation of the side effects of drugs used in treating hypertension should be done to rule out the possibility that they are causing insomnia.

Various herbs have been used in the treatment of high blood pressure, including hawthorn berries, buck wheat, marrow, lime flowers and mistletoe. Both the lime flowers and mistletoe also have sedative properties. The use of mistletoe is restricted to herbalists and medical practitioners. However, it's of great benefit in mild hypertension and anxiety states. It can be obtained in tincture form and the small amount of alcohol present in the tincture may also act as a mild sedative provided it's taken in the recommended dose. The small amount of alcohol won't do any damage to the liver or nervous system.

The use of mistletoe is also of benefit in patients suffering from arteriosclerosis, palpitations due to anxiety, headaches due to high blood pressure, shaking conditions of the elderly and some hysterical states.

Irritable bowel syndrome

The irritable bowel syndrome is a collection of symptoms consisting of abdominal pains, altered bowel function including constipation and diarrhoea, sometimes an excessive amount of mucus in the bowel, bowel wind and occasionally nausea. Anxiety and depression are commonly present in sufferers of irritable bowel.

Until proven otherwise, the irritable bowel syndrome is a food or chemical allergy. Anyone suffering from these symptoms should be carefully evaluated with respect to food and chemical sensitivities.

Dairy products are high on the list of foods aggravating the irritable bowel. Again, the stress foods are to be avoided. The best, and simplest, way of approaching the irritable bowel syndrome is to increase the amount of plant food (fruit and vegetables) in your diet. In particular, the green leafy vegetables are helpful. The most effective herbs in treating the irritable bowel syndrome include peppermint, slippery elm and plantago or psyllium seeds.

Peppermint oil has been shown scientifically to be very effective in the management of the irritable bowel syndrome and can be taken either as peppermint tea or more effectively as peppermint oil in capsule form. When taken regularly, many sufferers of the irritable bowel syndrome have found that peppermint is a life-enhancing herb.

The chronic low-grade pain of the irritable bowel syndrome makes many people's lives a misery. Restful sleep is often made extremely difficult. The use of these herbs will often settle the bowel and allow you a better quality of life and sleep.

Heart disorders

Sufferers of heart failure quite often find it difficult to lie flat in bed. If they do lie flat, their breathing becomes difficult because fluid tends to accumulate in the lungs. Therefore they have to sit up in bed at night and this can result in a poor night's rest and periods of insomnia.

To overcome this problem, these people are often given drugs such as digitalis and diuretics (tablets to remove fluid from the lungs and legs). The fluid tablets are usually taken in the morning to ensure that passing water is performed during the day. However, some people with heart disease find they frequently have to get up at night to pass urine. This can often be quite distressing.

The vitamin most commonly used to help to improve cardiac function is vitamin E. It can be taken in doses up to 2000 International Units per day. The use of these high doses of vitamin E is not advisable for people with heart disease complicated by high blood pressure.

However, there are usually no problems if vitamin E is taken by people with heart disease with normal blood pressure and the dose is increased slowly from 200 units per day up to 2000 units per day.

Herbs which are of benefit in treating heart disorders include hawthorn berries and garlic.

Herbs which are of benefit in treating heart disorders include hawthorn berries and garlic. Hawthorn berries contain chemicals called glycosides which help to strengthen and stimulate heart muscle. They can only be prescribed by a medical doctor or herbalist. Hawthorn berries can certainly augment the usual heart drugs.

Garlic has beneficial actions on the heart and blood vessel walls. Garlic is believed to reduce the amount of cholesterol and other fatty substances present in the blood. It also helps to lower blood pressure in people who have heart problems caused, or aggravated, by high blood pressure.

Garlic's antibacterial and antiviral properties are also of benefit in people with heart disease who are more prone to lung infections such as bronchitis, influenza and pneumonia. The routine use of garlic in people with heart disorders and weakened lungs is highly advisable. Not only does it help reduce the frequency and severity of these various illnesses, but it also helps to strengthen the person's constitution.

Hardening of the arteries

Hardening of the arteries, or arteriosclerosis, is a degenerative disorder of the arteries. It occurs with increasing age. The arteries become stiffer and contain more cholesterol than in younger people. Sometimes, calcium is deposited in the wall of the artery making it stiff and rigid, like a lead pipe. Consequently, the blood pressure tends to rise and less blood, oxygen and nutrients reach vital tissues including the brain, lungs and kidneys. With this reduction in blood flow, the functioning of these organs diminishes. Subtle changes occur in the organs which may result in mild to severe symptoms.

The elderly person suffering from insomnia may well benefit from an anti-stress program of supplements including vitamins, multiminerals, tryptophan and herbs.

The elderly person who suffers from insomnia may well benefit from the anti-stress program of supplements including vitamins, multiminerals, tryptophan and the various herbs. However, their general health may also be helped with the use of intravenous vitamin C, intramuscular vitamin B12 and folic acid, and a herb known as ginko biloba. This has been found to be useful in some degenerative diseases of the brain, including Parkinson's disease and arteriosclerosis. Vitamin B15, or pangamic acid, is another nutrient which helps to improve the oxygenation of the tissues including those of the central nervous system. It's used to improve muscle and lung function in athletes, greyhounds and racehorses. Pangamic acid should be tried if you are elderly, and suffer from hardening of the arteries with evidence of either poor blood flow to the brain or a poor heart.

Pregnancy

Sleep disorders may occur during pregnancy because of discomfort, particularly in the late stages of pregnancy as the large tummy is often difficult to place and remain comfortable. Sometimes, a flat cushion placed under the small of the back and a larger cushion behind the knees will allow a pregnant woman to recline in more comfort.

Calcium and magnesium are minerals which are safe to use during pregnancy and which may provide sedation. However, camomile tea is widely used in Europe and it does have sedative and relaxant properties. It's safe in pregnancy and can also help with the nausea and vomiting which occurs. Red raspberry leaf tea, or tablets, should be taken throughout pregnancy to prevent nausea and improve the labour and delivery.

> Camomile tea is safe to use in pregnancy and can also help with the nausea and vomiting which occurs.

Anaemia

People with anaemia are commonly extremely pale, tired, listless and unable to perform their normal everyday activities. The cause of their anaemia should be evaluated by a doctor and the cause eliminated or treated.

The causes of anaemia are too numerous to go into here. Some of the most common causes are blood loss through the bowel, by ulceration of the stomach or excessive alcohol or aspirin use. Very heavy periods are also a common cause of blood loss and anaemia. Some drugs can cause anaemia and it's well known that deficiencies of iron in the diet can contribute to or cause it. Pernicious anaemia is another form of anaemia which occurs as a result of vitamin B12 deficiency. Underlying blood disorders, leukaemia and cancer can be other reasons for the development of anaemia. Until the underlying cause for anaemia is properly evaluated, it's pointless doing anything else with such a patient suffering from insomnia.

However, it will be noticed that as soon as the anaemia is corrected, the pattern of insomnia changes and improvements in sleep occur. If the anaemia is due to an iron deficiency, one of the most common mineral deficiencies in the world, then not only will the anaemia improve but general levels of energy will increase accompanied by a greater feeling of wellbeing.

Parkinson's disease

This usually affects the elderly and is a degeneration of certain parts of the brain stem which results in a tremor and rigidity of the muscles with degeneration of the nervous system. Walking can become a shuffle and using a knife and fork or drinking from a cup can often be quite difficult.

Some drugs of course do help but they may also disrupt sleeping patterns.

The use of the Step-by-step summary of treatment on page 113 may slow the progression of Parkinson's disease.

Parkinson's disease itself may also contribute to insomnia. The use of the summary of treatment on pages 113–14 may slow the progression of Parkinson's disease.

The use of some adaptogenic and stimulating herbs in the early parts of the day can also help. Ginseng, Gotu kola and cayenne — either singly or in combination, used in the morning and at midday — can improve the condition over a period of three to six months.

Ginko biloba is another herb which has been shown to be of benefit, possibly by increasing blood flow through to the central nervous system. It's of probably more benefit with people who have Parkinson's disease secondary to arteriosclerosis. However, it's worth a trial of six weeks to three months.

An amino acid called D-L-phenylalanine may be of benefit to some people with Parkinson's disease. The usual dose is 250 milligrams twice daily. This can significantly improve walking ability, speech and depression in some people. However, there's usually no improvement in the tremor.

11

More about insomnia —
THE PSYCHOLOGICAL CAUSES

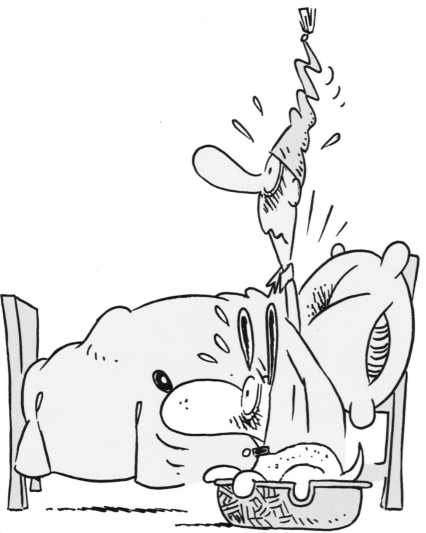

The mind and body

Your ability to adapt yourself to changing circumstances could be defined
as your level of intelligence. This ability to adapt is extremely important
for, without adaptation, we would suffer from continuous stress and its
associated anxieties and depressions.

Inside our own bodies are systems which also require adaptation and the most important one is the brain and nervous system. They must be able to adapt to rapid and subtle changes — both to our internal environment and to our external environment. The latter includes the physical environment such as heat and cold, hunger, angry people, loud noises and pollution.

The human body and brain have enormous potential for variation in various circumstances. When these functions are being adequately performed by the body and mind, we are usually in a state of what's called 'homeostasis'. Stress occurs if this natural balance, or homeostasis, is disturbed and our bodies and minds fail to adapt to changing circumstances. Some of the first symptoms which follow this maladaption are a change in appetite, feelings of inadequacy, loss of libido and insomnia.

CAROL'S STORY

Carol's job stress was such that she found that her relationship with her boyfriend had deteriorated and that she no longer wanted to see him, speak to him or have anything to do with him.

At only twenty-four, she found it increasingly difficult to cope as a director for a large advertising agency. 'My stress levels had become so great that I felt overwhelmed by severe anxiety, tension and at times suicidal feelings. I sought help from a psychiatrist which was sufficient to help me through my rough patches. However, my stress levels and other symptoms were such that I felt that I needed to do something more about them.'

It was discovered that her levels of vitamin C, B-complex and some minerals were low. She was prescribed the appropriate supplements and given daily injections of vitamin C and B for a week and then on a twice-weekly basis for another three weeks. 'I feel like a new woman,' she said. Her loving feelings for her boyfriend returned and she found she had the necessary creative energy to switch jobs in the same company.

Whenever she feels she is slipping back and not coping, Carol returns for the injection of vitamin C and B. She believes these have not only improved her physical ability to cope, but have also improved her mental capacity. 'They were lifesaving', she summed up at her last visit.

The sympathetic nervous system is responsible for, among other things, the 'fight or flight' response in which adrenaline (a hormone secreted by the adrenal glands) is released. Not only does this hormone prepare us for the 'fight or flight' response, but in excess it can also increase our levels of tension, anxiety, heart palpitations, sweating and general nervousness.

Thus, you can see that the nervous system influences the hormonal systems and these hormones can have wide-reaching effects on the body's activities. You certainly need adrenaline to function. But, too much in our bloodstream can be overstimulating and actually damaging to our cells and tissues.

Anxiety

Anxiety is a feeling of uncertainty and it may, or may not, have an obvious cause. Anxiety seems to be everywhere and is a normal part of our day-to-day living. It becomes serious when it's severe and is no longer a transient symptom. Chronic anxiety can be so disturbing that it stops normal activities and can result in excessive medical and psychiatric visits, expensive investigations and often futile hospitalisations.

Anxiety seems to be everywhere and is a normal part of our day-to-day living.

Anxiety may be the result of internal conflicts which have never been honestly resolved. Psychological symptoms of these conflicts include insecurity, dependency states, anger and hostility and concerns over power and control.

The symptoms of anxiety include physical and psychological changes. Tension, stress, fears, apprehensions, painful memories and poor concentration are frequent psychological symptoms.

Anxiety sufferers also produce, via the nervous system, such symptoms as heart palpitations, uncontrollable sweating, tremors and shakes, abdominal cramps, diarrhoea and frequency of urination. There are both psychological and physical causes for many people's anxiety. However, there are a number of good dietary approaches to the management of most anxiety problems.

The most common substances in your diet producing anxiety states are sugar, white flour products, caffeine, cola drinks and alcohol. Alcohol and caffeine both increase the amount of lactic acid in the blood and this particular acid is known to cause anxiety and tension states. Many people are also very sensitive to sugar.

Large quantities of sugar, which is probably one of the most highly refined substances we have in our diet, can cause derangements of our biochemistry. High concentrations of sugar are known to be toxic to brain cells.

For the anxiety sufferer, it's also important to rule out food and chemical allergies. The elimination of foods which can also act as stimulants and depressants is very important.

If you suffer from anxiety, follow the Step-by-step summary of treatment at the end of this book. Deficiencies or low levels of vitamin B in particular, can contribute to much anxiety and tension.

Vitamin B3, or niacinamide, has a very similar effect to the tranquillising drug diazepam and in fact, in animal studies, it's been shown to reduce the amount of conflict between animals, suppress aggressive behaviour, relax muscles and have a hypnotic or sleep-inducing action. This is similar to the minor tranquillising drugs used in medicine. The dose of niacinamide suggested is 250 to 500 milligrams three times a day.

Vitamin B6 in doses of 50 to 100 milligrams once or twice a day helps to reduce the amount of lactic acid in the blood. It also has other actions on the central nervous system to help relax it. The minerals calcium and magnesium are also extremely important in helping to stabilise the nervous system.

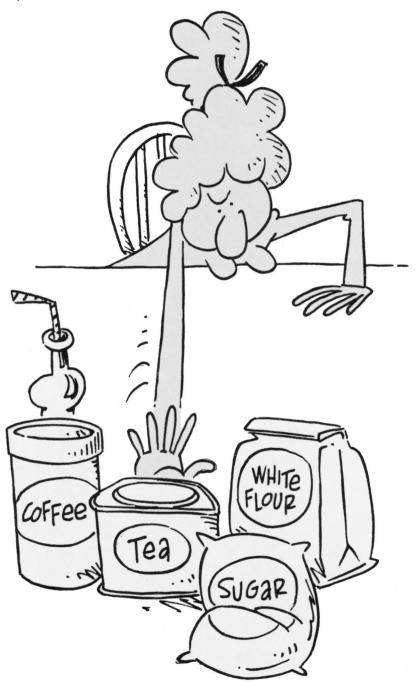

Another very important nutrient, which also helps with sleep is tryptophan. This has been used in a condition called the hyperventilation syndrome in which tense and anxious people over-breathe. This increased rate and depth of breathing is extremely distressing to the person who cannot control it. Tryptophan given in 500 to 1000 milligram doses three times a day with vitamin B6 can be very useful in this condition.

There is a very long list of herbs which can help the person with anxiety. Basically, these herbs are known as herbal relaxants which not only relax the mind and nervous system but also have an overall tranquillising effect on the body. It's important here to emphasise that some herbs may be more beneficial than others in this category. It depends on what other symptoms are occurring and disturbing the person.

Some herbs are more effective in relaxing the heart and vascular system, while others are good for settling down the irritable or nervous bowel, migraine headaches, nervous sweating and the premenstrual tension syndrome.

Relaxant herbs which can generally be used quite safely include camomile, valerian, passion flower, skullcap and vervain. There are of course stronger herbs in this category which have a more sedating effect but these are best handled by the qualified herbalist. These potent herbs include wild lettuce, ladies slipper and nightshade family.

Relaxant herbs which can generally be used quite safely include camomile, valerian, passion flower, scullcap and vervain.

Probably the best way of relieving muscle tension and anxiety is through exercise. In fact, yoga and tai chi are the best forms of exercise for anxiety sufferers. Only when absolutely necessary should a person with an anxiety state and tension resort to medical tranquillisers. These drugs only give temporary relief. They don't attempt to reach the core of the problem. There are nutrients for both strengthening and healing of the nervous system. Drugs will not do this.

Disorders of mood — mania and depression

DEPRESSION — CHEMICAL OR EMOTIONAL?

Depression is defined as a feeling of sadness and hopelessness, with a lowering of mood to a point where sometimes intense feelings of guilt occur. A person suffering from depression often has difficulty in speaking or putting their thoughts together. This includes the inability to concentrate on everyday tasks and to make normal everyday decisions.

With depression, there's a loss of interest in activities and a diminished involvement in both work and play. Usually, there are other physical complaints combined with a depressive type of illness. These can include a loss of appetite, a reduction in sexual drive, a marked increase or decrease in sleep and anxiety, headaches and inappropriate weight changes. In severe depression, of course, we have a risk of suicide as many depressed patients often contemplate ending it all.

There are many theories on the causes of depression. These include social factors, personality traits, genetic background, the loss of a loved one or favoured object or simply the personality of the depressed person using depression as a means of controlling others.

However, it's been my experience that most people suffering from depression can be helped by providing them with the basic building blocks for their nervous systems and bodily functions. These basic building blocks are amino acids, vitamins, minerals, trace elements, essential fatty acids and other naturally occurring compounds found in foods.

All of these substances should be available in your daily food intake. However, this is not always the case and many people in our society require nutrients in greater quantities than are available in their daily food to maintain the best health possible.

It's also been my experience that most depressed people have food allergies, food intolerances, chemical sensitivities, nutritional imbalances and low activity levels contributing greatly to their condition. Foods and chemicals may interrupt the sleep patterns of depressed people.

It's known that some food colourings are particularly stimulating to children. In adults, they may not show up as stimulants and produce hyperactivity (over-activity), but result in disturbance in sleep or in the inability to induce sleep.

It's well known that many adults will drink a glass of warm milk before retiring at night. Warm milk in a person allergic to milk can produce a state of fatigue and tiredness which will result in sleep. There's a theory that the tryptophan, an amino acid present in milk, may be the substance which induces sleep.

I don't believe it's only the tryptophan which induces sleep in many of these insomniacs, particularly in people with other diseases and disorders. Rather, it may be that the milk is contributing to their depression, arthritis, eczema, asthma, migraines and so on.

So, you can see that the inter-relationship between foods, diseases and daily activity is an extremely complex one. Milk may be of benefit to an insomniac, but in the majority of people it may actually be contributing to a degenerative disease.

As pointed out previously, the brain is a complex structure composed of chemicals derived from the diet. The function of the brain and the central nervous system is reliant on a balanced and regular supply of nutrients from the bloodstream. The proper management of a person's depression with diet and nutrient supplements will not only result in an improvement, or disappearance of depression, but an improvement in that person's life and lifestyle activities.

Sleep disorders are some of the most common symptoms of disorders of mood, or affective disorders, as they are sometimes called.

Sleep disorders are some of the most common symptoms of disorders of mood, or affective disorders, as they are sometimes known. Disorders of mood include depression and mania. It's usual for a person suffering from mood swings due to mania or depression to sleep more during the attacks of depression than when they are manic.

However, there's much variation to this pattern in each person. If a person does suffer from manic-depression, they often find it difficult to fall asleep and, when they do fall asleep, they often awake and find that their overall sleep time is reduced.

Generally, depressed people whether they have manic attacks or not, have a decreased total sleep time and the quality of the sleep they have is also poor. People suffering from pure depression often receive tricyclic anti-depressants, such as amitriptyline, at night.

These anti-depressants do have a sedating, as well as an anti-depressant, effect. However, long-term use can be harmful to overall health and natural sleeping patterns.

Lithium is a salt which is used for the treatment of mania and manic-depression and it also reduces REM sleep. Therefore, it can adversely affect the quality of a patient's sleep. However, some of these drugs can be lifesaving and, used in the short term, their harmful effects can be minimised.

While not neglecting some of the psychological factors in the aggravation of mania and manic depression, attention should be paid to the person's sensitivity to foods or food chemicals.

With depressive illness in particular, patients usually have sensitivities to many foods and to some chemicals in the environment. Removal of these foods often results in dramatic improvement. The Step-by-step summary outlined at the back of this book is the first step that a manic-depressive person with a sleep disorder should take.

Avoidance of stress foods is particularly important. The stress foods include sugar, white flour products, alcohol, tea, coffee, chocolate and cola drinks, all dairy foods, yeast and foods with chemical additives.

Supplementation with vitamin C and the bioflavonoids, B-complex vitamins and a broad spectrum mineral complex is essential. Generally, this group of patients requires the injection of some of the B-group and C vitamins to help achieve quick results. Although patients with mood disorders should be treated as individuals, there are some herbs which do help many of them. The adaptogenic herbs ginseng and Gotu kola are very important. In themselves, they don't have a direct effect on the disorder, but they assist the person's constitution to return to normal. They also facilitate the effects of other herbs and natural medicines used.

For the manic and over-active state, the use of the relaxant herbs mentioned in the section under anxiety is beneficial, in particular scullcap or passion flowers and valerian root. Hops is another herb which can be utilised in the manic state in combination with the others mentioned. However, if there is a risk of depression, then hops should be avoided.

Herbs suitable for use in depressive illnesses include some of the mild stimulants including cayenne, Gotu kola, vervain, rosemary and common oats.

It must be emphasised that in severe mood disorders, these herbs don't

Herbs suitable for use in depressive illnesses include some of the mild stimulants including cayenne, Gotu kola, vervain, rosemary and common oats.

act as symptom-controlling substances, but, over a period of three to six months, improvement can be seen in the person's psychological and physical constitution.

The most important vitamin in the mood disorders is niacinamide, or vitamin B3. The dosage can range from 1000 to 4000 milligrams per day. Vitamin C is also extremely important and should be given in doses of between 2000 to 8000 milligrams per day together with the bioflavonoids.

These are naturally occurring substances which are present in the peel of oranges and lemons and give these fruits their natural colouring. Some of the bioflavonoids have immune-enhancing properties while others have nervous system stimulating and regulating activities. They are particularly helpful in people who have mild to moderate depressive illnesses.

Unexpressed anger or resentment

These problems occur commonly in patients with psychological and psychiatric disturbances. They can result in substantial insomnia. The best form of management for a person with these outstanding symptoms is of course psychotherapy to talk out their underlying problems and to relieve themselves of inner conflicts.

However, some herbal and homeopathic remedies can benefit people with psychological and emotional disturbances. In particular, very sensitive patients with unresolved conflicts and unexpressed anger, resentment and fears can be helped by Bach flower remedies.

Remedies which may be of particular use include aspen, chicory, holly, impatiens, mustard, willow and a composite remedy called rescue remedy. The latter contains five individual Bach flower essences. These are impatiens, cherry plum, clematis, rock rose and star of Bethlehem. Rescue remedy, as its name suggests, can be used in times of an emergency and is particularly valuable when someone has had an emotional shock or trauma.

These remedies can be purchased through natural therapists or health food stores. Except for the rescue remedy, the others I have mentioned should be prescribed by a qualified natural therapist or medical practitioner experienced in the use of the Bach flower essences. They are extremely useful when used with properly selected patients.

Fear of dying while asleep

Fear of dying while asleep is not uncommon, especially in children who have experienced a death in the family.

This is not uncommon, especially in children who have experienced a death in the family. Quite often in young people suffering insomnia, this fear is maintained at a subconscious level. Again, a qualified psychiatrist should be consulted for further help with respect to these fears.

In addition, the use of the Bach flower remedies mentioned in the previous section and the relaxant herbs mentioned in the section on anxiety can play a supportive role in helping with these fears.

Sleep therapy, as outlined in Chapter 3, is sometimes invaluable in sleep disorders with children and can be used to allay their fears of dying while asleep. At some stage during the day or night, the child will fall asleep despite the problem of insomnia. It's during these periods of sleep that sleep therapy can be given.

The technique is easily learned and can be applied to all types of problems. For example, such things as nose picking, bed wetting, refusal to eat, tantrums and swearing can be stopped using sleep therapy. It's cheap and effective.

Schizophrenia

Many people with mild depression, anxiety and other psychological tension states, suffer sleep disorders at some time or another.

Many people with mild depression, anxiety and other psychological tension states suffer sleep disorders at some time or other.

However, schizophrenics often suffer very markedly in the degree of sleep disturbance that they endure. For example, in acute schizophrenia, the sleep disturbance is quite severe, often to the extent where the patient suffers from total insomnia. Frequently, the schizophrenic patient in remission, or the chronic long-term schizophrenic, doesn't have many sleep disorder complaints. Quite often, their brain wave patterns are normal. The anti-schizophrenic drugs, used in severe mental illness actually decrease what is known as 'sleep latency'. That is, there's a reduction in the time taken between going to bed and falling asleep. The anti-schizophrenic drugs also increase the overall sleep time and REM (Rapid Eye Movement) sleep. This is to the great benefit of the patient. The major drugs against schizophrenia, such as chloropromazine, if taken at bedtime, quite often obviate the need for hypnotics and sedatives in a schizophrenic patient with sleep disorders.

However, there are other ways to treat schizophrenia. In the early stages, where total or almost total insomnia occurs, supplementation with vitamin B complex, vitamin C and in particular tryptophan can be very beneficial. The dosage of tryptophan here may need to be 2000 milligrams taken in the late afternoon or early evening.

The avoidance of the B-complex vitamins after mid-afternoon is also important because vitamin B6 can act as a stimulant. However, nearly all schizophrenics will benefit from the use of these nutrients and the addition of zinc and vitamin B3 is of great advantage in long-term care.

It's been shown that the continued use of vitamin B3 can actually reduce the occurrence of attacks of schizophrenia and also the frequency and duration of hospital admissions. In fact, there are many patients in America and Australia who suffer from schizophrenia who lead normal lives taking large doses of vitamin B3 and vitamin C.

Some schizophrenics in the United States have responded so well to vitamin therapy that they have proceeded to become very successful psychiatrists themselves. As mentioned elsewhere in this book, vitamin B3 acts as a tranquilliser to the central nervous system in much the same way as some of the tranquillising drugs.

However, it doesn't have the same harmful side effects that many of the tranquillising drugs have. In fact, niacinamide, or vitamin B3 can actually improve mental and intellectual functioning as well as relieving anxiety and tension states. Although not as obvious, and strong, in effect as the drugs and some of the vitamins, the relaxant herbs can also help the nervous system of schizophrenia sufferers in the long term.

Importantly in schizophrenia, one must seek any underlying food allergy or chemical sensitivity. This is particularly so in patients who are reasonably well-controlled and who respond to vitamin B6 or pyridoxine.

It's interesting to note that many schizophrenics do have addictions to certain substances including tobacco (cigarette smoking), caffeine and some foods such as cows' milk, wheat, sugar and chocolate.

Their illness may have even been precipitated at a time when they were abusing substances like 'legal drugs' and the use of illegal drugs such as cocaine, marijuana or heroin. Schizophrenia starts as a brain sensitivity to either foods or chemicals, perhaps in early childhood,which results in behaviour, learning and psychological disorders.

If these disorders are not attended to, and the allergy removed, then to alter their way of feeling, people drift into the use of drugs or drug-like substances including sugar, tobacco, alcohol, caffeine and cola drinks.

These are substances which only temporarily remove the problem which inevitably becomes worse. This results in either a breakdown or the use of stronger and stronger drugs and medications.

This, in turn, results in further damage to the body's biochemistry with the resultant destruction or the excessive use of vitamins, minerals, amino acids, essential fatty acids and other nutrients. This is why the majority of people admitted to psychiatric institutions are suffering from one or more, and usually more, nutritional deficiencies.

The management of schizophrenia is therefore very complicated and it must be attended to by a qualified psychiatrist, preferably one who uses nutrition in his or her practice.

Step-by-step
SUMMARY OF TREATMENT

1. Remove or treat the known cause or causes of insomnia as they relate to you.

2. Change your bedroom so that it's warm, comfortable and peaceful.

3. Change your diet just slightly to start with by avoiding all 'stress' foods. This means none of the following:
- Sugar or sugar-containing products.
- Alcohol.
- Tea.
- Coffee.
- Chocolate.
- Cola-containing beverages and soft drinks.
- Tobacco
- Illegal drugs such as marijuana, cocaine and heroin.
- Chemically contaminated foods such as those with colourings, flavourings and preservatives (to which many people are allergic without realising it).

4. Slowly and gently increase your daily exercise. A walk for half-an-hour to one hour is excellent. Don't exercise after 7pm if possible. Perform light stretching exercises one hour before retiring.

5. Meditate or relax for at least twenty minutes twice a day in a chair or quiet place.

6. Most importantly supplement your diet with nutrients and herbs essential for a proper night's sleep and which are probably low in your foods due to processing and storage. The following nutrients should be tried in order:
- L-Tryptophan 400 to 4000 milligrams an hour before retiring, taken on an empty stomach. The usual dose is 800 to 1000 milligrams.
- Valerian root 500 to 1000 milligrams three times a day or 1000 milligrams at night. Persist with it for ten days.
- Magnesium orotate 400 milligrams. Two tablets in the evening.
- Niacinamide (Vitamin B3) 500 to 1000 milligrams, taken an hour before retiring.
- Passiflora 250 to 1000 milligrams three times a day or 500 to 1000 milligrams at night.
- Any other herbs listed in Chapter 8 which may suit your particular problem.

7. I personally recommend a product by the Vitaglow company called 'Naturest' which contains all of the above herbs and vitamins plus others in a balance suitable for most people. It contains, per tablet:

Valerian	100 mg
Passiflora	20 mg
Scullcap	20 mg
Vervain	25 mg
Magnesium oxide	160 mg
Calcium phosphate	130 mg
Vitamin B3	30 mg
Vitamin B6	15 mg
Vitamin C	50 mg
Tryptophan	200 mg

The usual dose is one to three tablets at night an hour before bed on an empty stomach and half-an-hour before any supper.

8. Persist with all of the above, especially the supplements, for at least four weeks. These supplements are not 'knock out' drugs. They may take a week or two to start their gentle, subtle sleep action. They are completely natural and generally safe to take over extended periods of time. If you have any problems, or questions, that this book hasn't answered, then contact a reputable nutritional doctor or natural therapist for further guidance.

9. It's always wise to take an additional supplement of vitamin C and the bioflavonoids daily, either in tablet or powdered form. The recommended dose for adults is 2000 to 4000 milligrams per day and for children 100 to 1000 milligrams per day from years one to ten. Vitamin C is as important as oxygen and water for life. It also promotes a feeling and appearance of well-being and slows down the ageing process.

10. Avoid all forms of chemical pollution including additives, especially sugar.

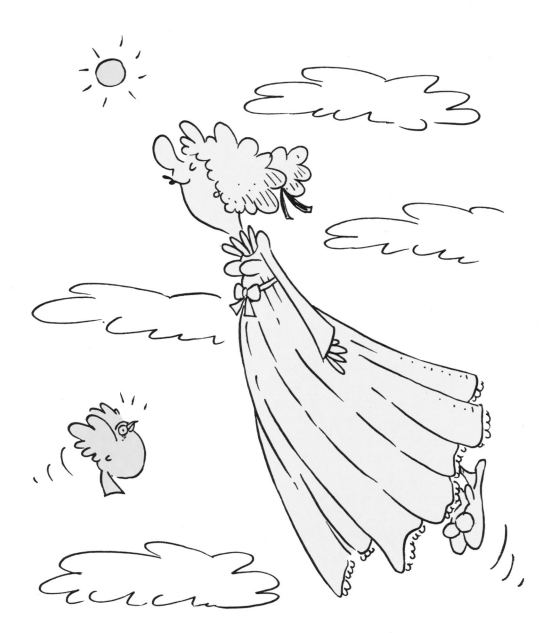

GLOSSARY

'Sleep that knits up the ravell'd sleave of care.'
SHAKESPEARE
(*Macbeth*, Act II, Scene II)

Adaptogenic herbs: Herbs which help maintain normal functioning in the face of acute or chronic stress.

Allergies: Food and chemical allergies are often a hidden cause of insomnia and other disorders. It's important to eliminate foods which can also act as stimulants and depressants — for example, sugar, white flour products, caffeine-containing drinks and alcohol. Tobacco is another substance to which insomniacs react allergically.

Amino acids: The building blocks of protein.

Amitriptyline: A tricyclic anti-depressant commonly given to depressed patients to help improve the quality of their sleep.

Anxiety: A major overlooked cause of poor sleep, often caused by a diet rich in sugar, white flour products, caffeine-containing drinks and alcohol.

Apnoea, sleep: A disorder characterised by periods in which the sleeper stops breathing, followed by loud snoring.

Arteriosclerosis: Degenerative change in the arteries associated with advancing age and resulting in a hardening of the walls of the arteries.

Asian ginseng: A relative of the rare and highly prized Panax ginseng renowned for its health-giving properties. Superior to the misnamed Siberian ginseng which is unrelated botanically to the Asian and Panax.

Avena sativa: see Oats.

Bach flowers: Fluid essences containing minute amounts of flower extracts and used to treat minor emotional disorders. They include aspen, chicory, holly, impatiens, mustard, willow and a composite remedy called rescue remedy. The latter contains five individual Bach flower essences. These are impatiens, cherry plum, clematis, rock rose and star of Bethlehem. Also see Rescue Remedy.

Barbiturates: Medical drugs used to sedate. They are very habit-forming and are rarely used nowadays.

Benzodiazepines: A family of drugs commonly known as minor tranquillisers. They include Valium and Serepax.

Bioflavonoids: Naturally occurring substances which are present in the peel of oranges and lemons and give these fruits their natural colouring. Some of the bioflavonoids have immune-enhancing properties while others have nervous system stimulating activities. They are particularly helpful for people who have mild depressive illness.

Biotin: A member of the vitamin B complex, a deficiency of which can cause dermatitis, depression and anaemia.

Broad spectrum mineral complex: A tablet containing all of the important minerals including calcium, magnesium, zinc, manganese, chromium, molybdenum, potassium, copper and iron.

Caffeine: A chemical in tea, coffee and cola drinks which is addictive and can cause headaches, pain, anxiety, tension, insomnia and palpitations. Withdrawal of caffeine leads to lethargy, depression, headaches and muscle pain.

Calcium: A mineral which is very important, together with magnesium, in helping stabilise the nervous system.

Camomile: A herb, the flowers of which are used for the relief of insomnia. It is particularly useful for children.

Cataplexy: Sudden loss of muscle tone at times of extreme emotion. Loss of consciousness usually does not occur.

Cayenne (red pepper chillies): A heating and stimulating herb used to increase circulation and to 'flush out' diseased tissue.

Chloral hydrate: A drug used to rapidly induce sleep.

Chlorpramazine: A major drug in the treatment of schizophrenia and other mental illness which, if taken at bed time, quite often obviates the need for hypnotics and sedatives in a schizophrenic with sleep disorders.

Choline: A mild (natural) sedative, this is a member of the vitamin B complex which is important for the proper functioning of nerves.

Circulatory stimulants: Horseradish, ginger or cayenne (red pepper chillies) stimulate blood flow into diseased tissues and thus aid people whose illness is made worse by cold weather. For example, arthritis and respiratory infections.

Clematis: A flower used in the Bach remedies for indifference and dreaminess.

Coxsackie B virus: A virus of the gastrointestinal tract which can cause severe illness and which may result in the post-viral-fatigue syndrome if the person was not in reasonably good health at the time of the infection.

Damiana: A herb from Mexico useful in depression and sexual inadequacy due to psychological problems.

Diazepam: A tranquilliser-sedative with muscle relaxant properties. It's habit-forming and available under a number of different brands.

D-L-phenylalanine: Probably the most important nutrient substance in the relief of pain, this amino acid occurs in the diet and stops the breakdown of enkephalins in the central nervous system, which means we tend to feel less pain.

Efamol: See Evening Primrose Oil.

Electro-convulsive therapy: An electric shock given to anaesthetised patients suffering from life-threatening depression. It's effective in extreme circumstances and safe in the right hands.

Endorphins: The brain's naturally occurring pain-controlling substances. They are inhibited by excessive caffeine.

Enkephalins: Substances produced by brain cells to stop pain. Enkephalins are produced in the presence of copper. The production of enkephalins is reduced if you are copper deficient, either through not consuming adequate copper in the diet or by using large quantities of zinc and iron supplements.

Epidemic neuromyasthenia: See Post-viral Fatigue Syndrome (PVFS).

Epstein Barr virus: A virus associated with the post-viral fatigue syndrome. It causes a malignancy of the lymph glands in Africans.

Evening primrose oil: An oil from the evening primrose plant which contains an essential fatty acid called gamma linolenic acid (GLA). This substance is important in many immunological actions in the body. It's effective for many allergic conditions including severe eczema, asthma and is of benefit in some disorders of the immune system including rheumatoid arthritis.

Feverfew: A herb which blocks inflammatory substances in the body. It was shown to be more effective in treating inflammatory conditions, including arthritis, than some of the drugs commonly used.

Folic acid: A member of the vitamin B complex, a deficiency of which results in anaemia, memory deterioration and apathy.

Gentian: A herb who's bitter root stimulates digestion and is anti-inflammatory. It can be used to help people with insomnia who have digestive disorders and chronic inflammatory diseases.

Ginseng: See Asian Ginseng.

Ginger: A heating herb useful in treating diseases of the lungs, intestinal 'nerves' and spasms and motion sickness.

Ginko biloba: A herb useful in some degenerative diseases of the brain, including Parkinson's disease and arteriosclerosis.

Gotu kola: An Indian herb of great benefit in nervous and mental disorders. It's used in leprosy and other infectious diseases.

Grenadille: The homeopathic remedy made from the flower which produces the well-known passionfruit. Its specific use in herbal medicine is as an hypnotic herb for the treatment of insomnia. However, it's also of benefit to people suffering from heart palpitations, asthma, nerve pains or neuralgia and, in some cases, Grand Mal epilepsy. Grenadille is also called maypop and passion flower.

Holly: A Bach flower remedy useful for sufferers of jealousy, hatred and envy.

Hops: A herb useful for insomnia, excitability, nerve pain and mucous colitis. It's especially useful for restlessness, but it may make some depressive patients worse.

Horseradish: A heating herb useful in lung and kidney infections and sinus disorders. It should not be used if there is low thyroid activity.

Hypersomniacs: People, often over-weight, who complain of falling asleep daily several times a week. The only thing which may help them is a general improvement in lifestyle, including increasing daytime activity and exercise programs, diet changes to reduce weight and the use of the anti-stress supplements.

Hyperventilation syndrome: A condition in which tense and anxious people over-breathe. This increased rate and depth of breathing is extremely distressing to the sufferer who cannot control it. Tryptophan given in 500 to 1000 milligram doses three times a day with vitamin B6 can be very useful in this condition.

Hypoglycaemia: A condition in which the body's blood sugar falls below a certain level. The effect is that the low blood sugar level starves the brain and other body organs of essential fuel. This can result in a multitude of symptoms often classed as psychosomatic or hypochondriacal.

Immunoglobulin G: A special solution extracted from human blood which contains high levels of antibodies .. the important factors in fighting infections in the blood.

Impatiens: A Bach flower remedy useful in treating people with emotional disorders including mental stress, irritability, impatience and impulsiveness.

Inactivity-pseudo-hibernation-syndrome: A term used by this author to describe severe fatigue, dullness and insomnia caused by an almost totally inactive lifestyle.

Inositol: A member of the vitamin B complex which has mild sedating properties and also helps to lower cholesterol.

Irritable bowel syndrome: The irritable bowel syndrome is characterised by abdominal pain, diarrhoea or constipation, bowel mucous, wind and sometimes nausea. The causes of the irritable bowel syndrome such as allergies and nutritional deficiencies are often similar to the causes of insomnia, anxiety and depression.

Lactic acid: An acid found in body tissues which, in high concentrations, can cause anxiety. Sources are excessive exercise, milk, sugar, and lactose.

Ladies slipper: A herb also known as nerve root. It acts as a tonic to the nervous system by sedating it. It also helps anxiety neurosis and insomnia during convalescence.

Lemon balm: An effective herb for children's insomnia. It has the benefit of being a pleasant-tasting drink.

Lime flowers: A herb useful for insomnia, children's irritability and fever management.

Lithium: A salt used for the treatment of mania and manic depression, it also reduces REM sleep. Therefore, it can adversely affect the quality of sleep. However, some of these drugs can be lifesaving and, used in the short term, their harmful effects can be minimised.

Lobelia: A herb, also known as Indian tobacco, very effective in relieving asthma, bronchitis and some nervous disorders. Its use is restricted to qualified practitioners.

Magnesium: A mineral which is very important, together with calcium, in helping stabilise the nervous system. Magnesium helps some twitches, tremors, muscle aches, depression, irritability, insomnia and hyperactivity.

Maypop: See Grenadille.

Melatonin: A hormone secreted by the pineal gland in the centre of the brain. It's important in pigment deposition in skin, sleep-wake cycles, sexuality and mood swings related to inadequate sunlight.

Mistletoe: A parasitic herb which grows on trees such as fruit trees, oak, poplar and wattle. It is useful in overactive heart conditions, high blood pressure, some cancers and nervous tension.

Myalgic Encephalomyelitis (ME): See Post-viral Fatigue Syndrome (PVFS).

Narcolepsy: An uncontrollable desire to sleep. According to most authorities, the cause is unknown. However, anecdotal reports include patients cured by the removal of food chemical sensitivities.

Neuralgia: Nerve pains, especially in the face.

Neurotransmitter: A chemical messenger which travels from one nerve cell or group in the brain to others, directing their function and activities. Amino acids from protein foods commonly act as neurotransmitters.

Niacin: Vitamin B3. There are two forms of vitamin B3. Nicotinic acid is useful in reducing cholesterol, but causes severe flushing in high doses. Niacinamide is sedating but doesn't reduce cholesterol.

NREM Sleep: Deep sleep, that is, the periods of sleep when rapid eye movement doesn't occur.

Oats, common: A restorative herb for the nervous system.

Pangamic acid: See vitamin B15.

Paradoxical insomnia: Insomnia caused by so-called hypnotic or sedating drugs initially prescribed to help anxiety, depression or insomnia. They start working in an opposite way to that originally intended.

Passion flower: A herb useful for insomnia and painful conditions. It must be used for a few weeks to obtain the full benefits.

Peppermint oil: This has been scientifically shown to be very effective in the management of the irritable bowel syndrome and can be taken either as peppermint tea or more effectively as peppermint oil in capsule form.

Peptide: A small fragment of a protein molecule. See Sleep chemicals.

Phytotherapy: Plant therapy or the treatment of disorders using herbs and plants.

Pineal gland: A pea-size gland situated in the centre of the brain. This gland is responsible for the secretion of hormones. Its activity depends on the amount of light falling on the eyes. The pineal gland secretes melatonin — important in pigment deposition in skin.

Plantago or psyllium seeds: A herb useful in treating bowel disease, irritable colon and constipation.

Post-Viral Fatigue Syndrome (PVFS): This is another way of describing extreme muscle fatigue following an acute viral illness such as influenza, hepatitis or glandular fever. The syndrome not only includes severe fatigue, which is the cardinal symptom, but many other symptoms as well. Muscle fatigue, especially following minor exertion, is the main symptom but muscle aches and pains are also common together with concentration difficulties, short-term memory loss, anxiety, depression, joint pains, headaches, swelling of the glands and intermittent fevers. The depression associated with this syndrome can be linked to severe insomnia and, at times, over-sleeping at the wrong time of the day. The sleep-wake cycle therefore appears to be interfered with or interrupted in some way. Also called 'myalgic encephalomyelitis', 'the Royal Free disease'; 'the Iceland disease'; 'epidemic neuromyasthenia', 'chronic fatigue syndrome', and, inappropriately, 'the yuppie flu'.

Potassium: A mineral normally occurring in the diet. Deficiencies of potassium can cause muscle fatigue, cramps, apathy and heart disorders.

Pyridoxine: See Vitamin B6.

Rapid Eye Movement (REM) sleep: The dreaming phase of sleep. REM sleep is very important for mental and physical rejuvenation and repair. Babies have REM sleep for about fifty per cent of the time whereas adults have it for about ten to twenty per cent.

Reactive functional hypoglycaemia: The disease caused by consumption of refined carbohydrates, including alcohol and especially sugar, often resulting in anxiety, depression and sleep disorders.

Rescue remedy: A combination of five Bach flowers. As its name suggests, it can be used in times of emergency and is particularly valuable when someone has had an emotional shock or trauma.

Rock rose: A Bach flower remedy to help panic, fear and terror.

Rosemary: A herb useful for depression, migraines, liver disorders and nervous tension.

Salicylates: Aspirin-like compounds. See Willow.

Scullcap: A herb for sedation, nervous exhaustion and possibly of help in epilepsy.

Sedatives: Drugs, or herbal medicines, used to reduce nervous activity and useful in helping to induce sleep.

Serotonin: A chemical messenger, or neurotransmitter, very important for the induction and maintenance of the sleep state. Formed in the brain from the amino acid tryptophan.

Sleep chemicals: These are chemicals produced in our own bodies which may be responsible for putting us to sleep and keeping us that way. A peptide (a small fragment of a protein molecule) called Delta-sleep-inducing-peptide (DSIP) has been isolated from sleeping animals. When DSIP is injected into the brain of awake animals, they become drowsy and the brain waves become 'sleepy'.

Sleep latency: The time taken between lights out and a moderate depth of sleep.

Sleep therapy: A very effective form of hypnotherapy given to a sleeping child by an informed parent.

Slippery elm: A herb of great benefit for treating disorders of the gullet, stomach, duodenum and intestines. It soothes the entire digestive system and is used in treating ulcers, indigestion, hiatus hernia, diarrhoea and some cases of irritable colon. It is thus a very effective way of promoting sleep by removing pain and discomfort.

Squaw vine: A herbal tonic for the nervous system, especially when it affects the reproductive system. It's good for painful periods and for relaxing the uterus during child birth.

St John's wort: A herb useful for irritability and anxiety, especially in the presence of neuralgia and fibrositis.

Star of Bethlehem: A Bach flower remedy for emotional shock.

Stress foods: Sugar, white flour products, alcohol, tea, coffee, chocolate and cola drinks, all dairy foods and yeast can all be implicated in sleep disturbances with susceptible individuals. Foods containing any chemical additives such as colourings, flavourings and preservatives should be regarded as stress foods.

Stress-tension-fatigue syndrome: A collection of syndromes which are part of a vicious cycle in which mental stress is made worse by the very symptoms it produces.

Sugar: A potent cause of insomnia and sleep problems. Sugar is highly damaging, even in small doses over a long time.

Tricyclic anti-depressants: Drugs used to treat depression but having some sedating side effects.

Tryptophan: An amino acid which is a basic building block found in protein. It's converted in the brain to serotonin and vitamin B3. Serotonin is the brains chemical messenger or neurotransmitter, which is responsible for the sleep-wake cycles of our body. Tryptophan is relaxing and sleep-inducing.

Valerian: A most useful non-addictive herb for anxiety and insomnia. It's probably considered to be the number one herb for helping restore the insomniac's nervous system.

Vervain: Also known as verbena, this is a useful herb for insomniacs who have asthma, migraine, fevers, liver disorders and for lactating mothers who wish to boost their milk productivity.

Vitamin B3: Also called niacinamide and nicotinic acid, this has a very similar effect to diazepam and, in fact, in animals it's been shown to reduce the amount of conflict between animals, suppress aggressive behaviour, relax muscles and have a hypnotic or sleep-inducing action very similar to the minor tranquillising drugs used in medicine. The dose of niacinamide suggested is 250 to 500 milligrams three times a day.

Vitamin B6: Also known as pyridoxine, in doses of 50 to 100 milligrams once or twice a day, it helps reduce the amount of lactic acid in the blood, anxiety and the symptoms of pre-menstrual tension. Vitamin B6 also has other actions on the central nervous system to help relax it. The minerals calcium and magnesium are also extremely important in helping stabilise the nervous system in conjunction with vitamin B6.

Vitamin B15: Also known as pangamic acid, this is another nutrient which helps to improve the oxygenation of the tissues including the central nervous system. It's used to improve muscle and lung function in athletes, greyhounds and racehorses. Pangamic acid should be tried by elderly people who suffer from hardening of the arteries with evidence of either poor blood flow to the brain or a poor heart.

Vitamin D: A fat-soluble vitamin necessary to prevent rickets. Low levels may result in rheumatic pains, exhaustion and menopausal symptoms.

Vitamin E: A fat-soluble vitamin which, if deficient, can cause fatigue, fitful sleep, insomnia, destruction of red cells, muscle wasting, liver and kidney damage, sensitivity to chemicals, vascular disease and menopausal symptoms.

Wild lettuce: A herb reserved for severe insomnia and of particular benefit in very restless, excitable children suffering from irritable coughs.

Willow: A herb containing salicylates (aspirin-like compounds) useful in rheumatic, arthritic, and other inflammatory pain.

Wintergreen: A herb effective in pain relief, especially for rheumatic and arthritic conditions and the pain associated with muscle disorders.

Yuppie flu: See Post-viral Fatigue Syndrome.

Zinc: Required by the skin, hormone glands, brain, pancreas and lymph glands for proper functioning. Low zinc levels are associated with a high incidence of severe infections. Rich natural sources of zinc include red meat, fish, pumpkin seeds, sunflower seeds and oysters. Care is advised with oysters because they may contain heavy metals.

FURTHER READING

Nutrition and Vitamin Therapy — Dr Michael Lesser M.D., Bantam, New York, 1980.

Nutritional Influences On Illness — Dr. Melvyn R. Werbach, Third Line Press, Tarzana, California, 1987.

A-Z of Natural Health — Judy Jacka, Lothian, Melbourne, 1987.

Psychodietetics — Dr. E. Cheraskin, Bantam, New York, 1977.

Manage Your Pain — Dr. Leonard Rose with Peter Fitzgerald, Angus & Robertson, Australia, 1987.

Food Chemical Sensitivity — Dr. Robert Buist, Harper & Row, Sydney, 1986.

British Herbal Pharmacopoeia — British Herbal Medicine Association, Great Britain, 1983.

Nutritional Medicine — Dr. Stephen Davies, Pan Books, London, 1987.

Nutrients — Dr. Ian Brighthope with Peter Fitzgerald (Biocentres),published in the USA by Keats Publishing, Inc, as The AIDS Fighters, 1987.

Food For Thought — Maureen Minchin, Unwin, Australia, 1986.

Peace of Mind — Dr. Ian Gawler, Hill of Content, Australia, 1987.

INDEX